Practical Manual and Workbook of HISTOLOGY

Third Edition

As per the latest NMC Guidelines | Competency Based Medical Education (CBME) Curriculum under Graduate Medical Education Regulation

Name: ______________________________

Roll No. : ______________ University Registration No. : ______________

Date of Admission: ______________________________

Permanent Address: ______________________________

E-mail ID: ______________ Batch: ______________

Mobile No. : ______________________________

Review Comment

In *Practical Manual and Workbook of Histology*, students find the solutions to their question, how to draw, 'What to draw', What to focus on. After studying histology slides under microscope. The micro-photographs provided in the manual give the actual features for reference.

I congratulate the authors for bringing out the third edition that includes CBME curriculum

Dr Arun V Kulkarni MBBS, MD
Professor, Department of Anatomy
SDM College of Medical Sciences and Hospital
Shri Dharmasthala Manjunatheshwara University, Dharwad

- It is a very useful workbook for undergraduate medical and paramedical students.
- The book includes neatly hand-drawn diagrams with labelling, the key features to identify the slides, enabling the students for easy learning and quick recapitulation during assessment.
- The book covers all the slides with the competency numbers according to CBME curriculum and also more clinical correlation incorporated.

Dr Shilpa M Bhimalli
Professor
Department of Anatomy
KAHER'S JN Medical College, Belagavi

Practical Manual and Workbook of HISTOLOGY

Third Edition

As per the latest NMC Guidelines | Competency Based Medical Education (CBME) Curriculum under Graduate Medical Education Regulation

Veena V Kulkarni
MBBS, MD

Professor and Head
Department of Anatomy
SDM College of Medical Sciences and Hospital
Shri Dharmasthala Manjunatheshwara University
Dharwad, Karnataka

Rakesh Kumar
MSc (Medical Anatomy)

Assistant Professor
Department of Anatomy
Zydus Medical College and Hospital
Dahod, Gujarat

CBSPD

CBS Publishers & Distributors Pvt Ltd

New Delhi • Bengaluru • Chennai • Kochi • Kolkata • Lucknow • Mumbai
Hyderabad • Jharkhand • Nagpur • Patna • Pune • Uttarakhand

Practical Manual and Workbook of

HISTOLOGY

ISBN: 978-93-5466-889-0

Third Edition: 2025
Reprint: **2026**
First Edition: 2021
Reprint: 2021
Second Edition: 2022
Reprint: 2023, 2024

Published by Satish Kumar Jain and produced by Varun Jain for
CBS Publishers & Distributors Pvt Ltd
4819/XI Prahlad Street, 24 Ansari Road, Daryaganj, New Delhi 110 002, India
Ph: 011-23289259, 23266838 Website: www.cbspd.com
e-mail: delhi@cbspd.com

Corporate Office: 204 FIE, Industrial Area, Patparganj, Delhi 110 092, India
Ph: 011-49344934 Fax: 011-49344935 e-mail: publishing@cbspd.com; publicity@cbspd.com

Branches

- **Bengaluru:** Seema House 2975, 17th Cross, KR Road, Banasankari 2nd Stage, Bengaluru 560 070, Karnataka, India
  Ph: +91-80-26771678/79 Fax: +91-80-26771680 e-mail: bangalore@cbspd.com
- **Chennai:** 18/8B, Subbarayan Street, Shenoy Nagar, Chennai 600 030, Tamil Nadu, India
  Ph: +91-44-42032115, 45022115 e-mail: chennai@cbspd.com
- **Kochi:** 42/1325, 1326, Power House Road, Opposite KSEB, Kochi 682018, Kerala, India
  Ph: +91-484-4059061–67 Fax: +91-484-4059065 e-mail: kochi@cbspd.com
- **Kolkata:** 147, Hind Ceramics Compound, 1st Floor, Nilgunj Road, Belghoria, Kolkata 700056, West Bengal, India
  Ph: +91-33-25633055/56 e-mail: kolkata@cbspd.com
- **Lucknow:** Basement, Khushnuma Complex, 7 Meerabai Marg (behind Jawahar Bhawan), Lucknow 226001, UP, India
  Ph: +91-522-4000032 e-mail: tiwari.lucknow@cbspd.com
- **Mumbai:** PWD Shed, Gala No. 25/26, Ramchandra Bhatt Marg, Next JJ Hospital Gate No. 2, Opp. Union Bank of India, Noorbaug, Mumbai 400009, Maharashtra, India
  Ph: +91-22-66661880/89 e-mail: mumbai@cbspd.com

Representatives

• **Gujarat** • **Hyderabad** • **Jharkhand** • **Nagpur** • **Patna** • **Pune** • **Uttarakhand**

For trade terms please contact customercare@cbspd.com
For general enquiries please contact info@cbspd.com

Printed at Sriprints & Sales, Delhi, India

Foreword

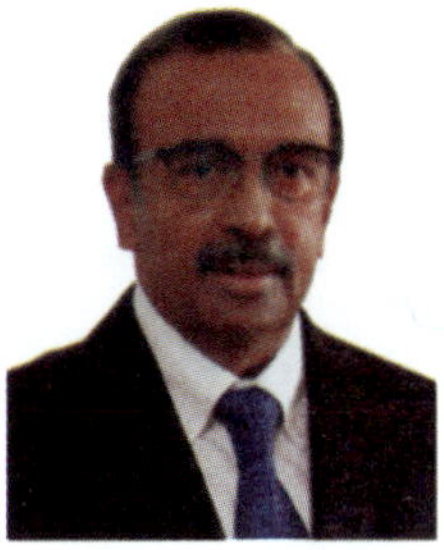

I am extremely happy to know that the third edition of *Practical Manual and Workbook of Histology* is coming up.

Authors have taken efforts to include pictures of histological slides along with the schematic diagrams that will help the students to understand and draw diagrams in an easier and simpler way.

Also in this edition frequently asked questions have been incorporated as per CBME curriculum with emphasis on clinical histoloy.

This book will certainly benefit the students. It will create interest in the subject, enhance their knowledge and build a firm foundation for their medical career in future.

Niranjan

Dr Niranjan Kumar
Hon'ble Vice Chancellor
Shri Dharmasthala Manjunatheshwara University
Dharwad, Karnataka

Preface to the Third Edition

The *Practical Manual and Workbook of Histology* was conceived with a clear vision to address the challenges faced by medical, dental, and paramedical students in accurately replicating histological diagrams from various, often similar-looking, slides.

Recognizing that schematic diagrams can differ significantly from the natural appearance of slides under the microscope, we have meticulously compiled photographs of histological slides from our department and paired them with hand-drawn schematic diagrams organized system-wise. This approach ensures that students can more easily correlate the schematic representations with the actual microscopic images they will encounter.

In this updated third edition, we have gone a step further by including key features, detailed descriptions of the slides, applied histology, and relevant competency numbers. Moreover, to better serve our students, we have added relevant questions frequently asked in examinations, enabling a more comprehensive and exam-oriented study experience.

Our sincere effort is to make this manual as student-friendly as possible, fostering a deeper interest and understanding of histology, and aiding students in drawing accurate diagrams in their practical histology record books.

We warmly welcome valuable comments and suggestions that will help us to continually improve this book in future editions.

We would like to humbly acknowledge Dr Subhash K Deshpande, Professor, Department of Anatomy, and Dr Arun V Kulkarni, Professor, Department of Anatomy, SDM College of Medical Sciences and Hospital, Dharwad, Karnataka, for their support and guidance.

Our heartfelt thanks go to all our departmental colleagues and technicians for their kind cooperation.

Veena V Kulkarni
Rakesh Kumar

Preface to the First Edition

The *Practical Manual and Workbook of Histology* was conceptualized keeping in mind the difficulties encountered by the medical, dental and paramedical students while replicating the diagrams from various similar looking histology slides.

The schematic diagrams would differ to some extent from the natural appearance of the slides under the microscope. To resolve these challenges we have compiled the pictures of histological slides available in our department with handdrawn schematic diagrams system wise. Also a few key features necessary to identify the slides have been included.

It is our sincere effort to make this manual student-friendly so that they develop interest in understanding and drawing the histology diagrams in their practical histology record book.

We are welcome to valuable comments and suggestions which will help us to further improve our book in the future.

We would like to humbly acknowledge Dr Subhash K Deshpande, Head, Department of Anatomy, SDM College of Medical Sciences and Hospital, Karnataka, for all his support and guidance.

We sincerely thank all our departmental colleagues and technicians for their kind co-operation.

Veena V Kulkarni
Rakesh Kumar

Contents

Index of Competencies

1 Microscope

LIGHT MICROSCOPE

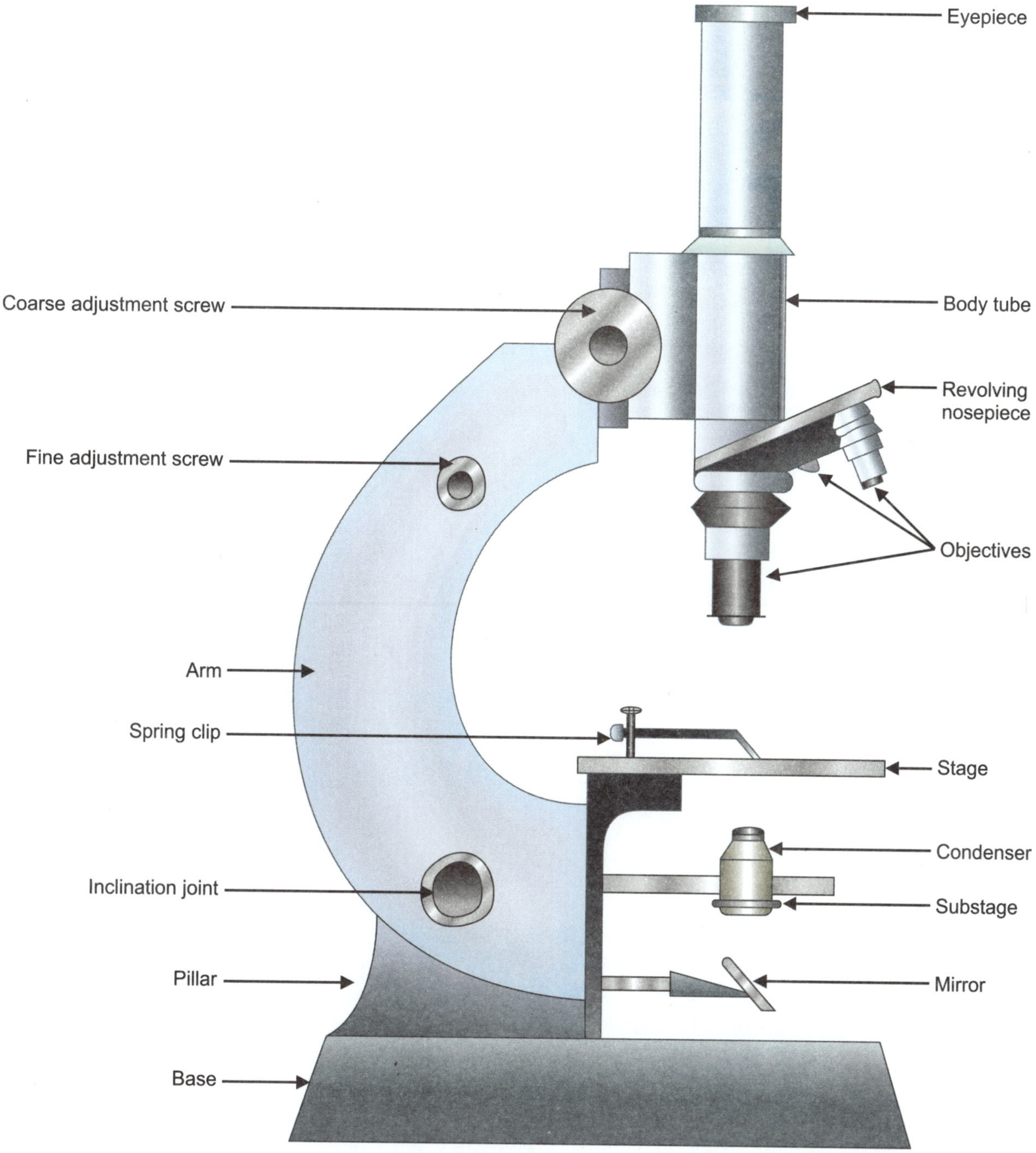

Figures/Notes

Figures/Notes

2 Epithelial Tissue (AN 65.1, 65.2)

- Epithelium is one of the basic tissues of the body that covers or lines all body surfaces, cavities and tubes.
- Epithelial cells are bound to adjacent cells by various types of cell junctions and all epithelia are supported by a basement membrane.
- Basic functions of epithelia based on their location includes providing protection, acting as mechanical barrier, involved in absorption, secretion and sensory perception.
- Epithelia are classified based on layers of cells as—simple epithelium with only one layer of cells, stratified epithelium with two or more layers of cells, pseudostratified epithelium and transitional epithelium.
- Epithelia are classified based on shape of cells facing towards free surface as squamous epithelium made up of flat cells, cuboidal epithelium made up of cells with equal height and width, columnar epithelium composed of cells with more height than width.
- Pseudostratified epithelium is simple epithelium since all the cells rest on basement membrane. The nuclei of these cells are disposed at different levels thus creating the illusion of stratification.
- Apical or luminal surface of epithelial cells may incorporate three main types of specialization—cilia which are actively motile structures, microvilli—the shorter projections of plasma membrane, stereocilia are non-motile extremely long microvilli.
- Epithelium primarily involved in secretion is often arranged into structures called glands (glandular epithelia). Glands are merely invagination of epithelial surfaces into the underlying structure.
- Glands are broadly classified as exocrine glands, which release their secretions through the duct and endocrine glands, which have no duct system and release their secretions into the bloodstream.
- Exocrine glands are classified: 1. based on their duct system into simple (unbranched) glands and compound (branched) glands, 2. based on secretory component into tubular or acinar (alveolar).

Applied Aspects of Epithelial Tissue

1. Epithelial cell tumor: It is a swelling that occurs due to excessive proliferation of cells which can be benign or malignant when it is termed as carcinoma.
2. Metaplasia: It is abnormal replacement of one type of epithelium by another type of epithelium on exposure to certain factors like loss of cilia from the epithelium of trachea on exposure to cigarette smoke.

SIMPLE EPITHELIUM

Simple Squamous Epithelium

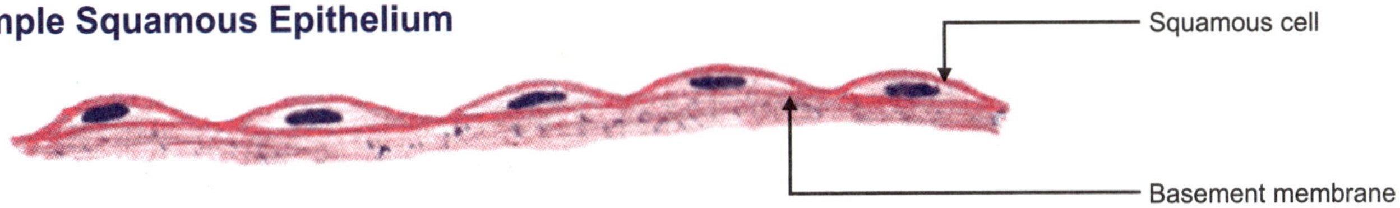

Examples

- Alveoli of lung and endothelium of blood vessels

Simple Cuboidal Epithelium

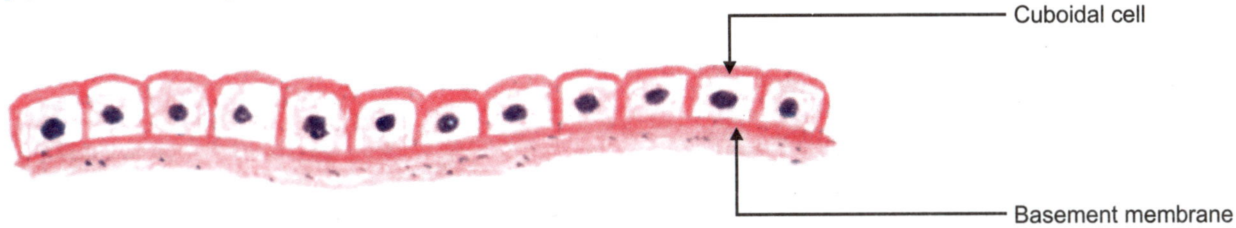

Examples

- Follicles of thyroid gland
- Ducts of exocrine glands

Simple Columnar Epithelium

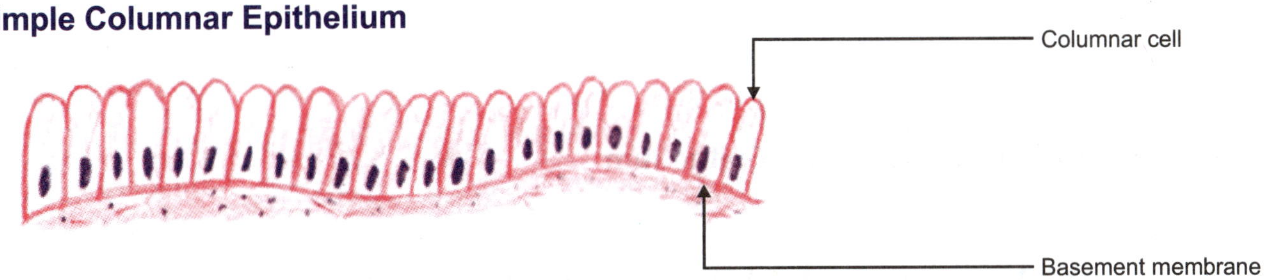

Examples

- Small intestine
- Uterus

APICAL SURFACE MODIFICATION OF COLUMNAR EPITHELIUM

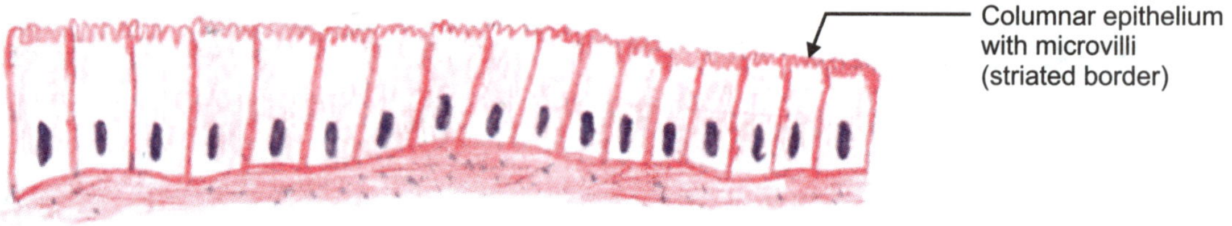

Examples

- Duodenum, jejunum and ileum

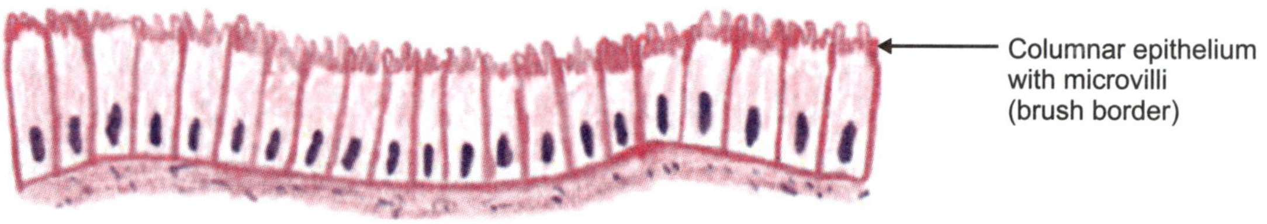

Examples

- Gallbladder and PCT of kidney

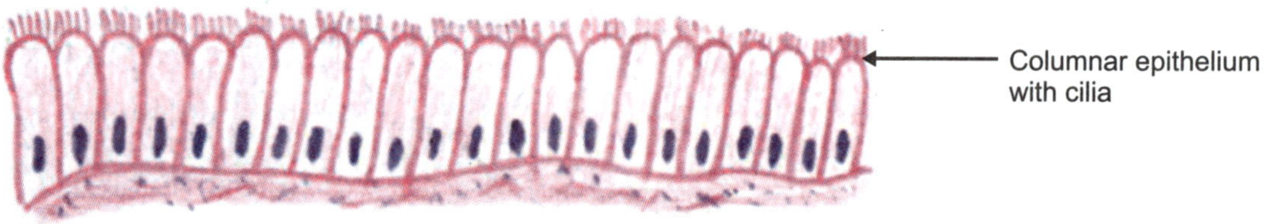

Examples

- Fallopian tube and auditory tube

Pseudostratified Ciliated Columnar Epithelium

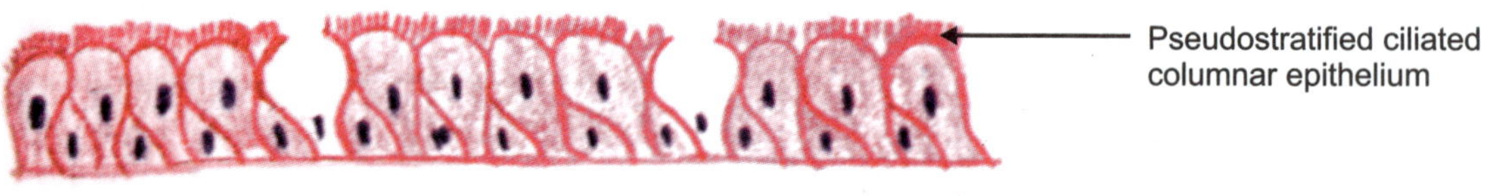

Examples

- Trachea and bronchi

Figures/Notes

STRATIFIED SQUAMOUS NON-KERATINIZED EPITHELIUM

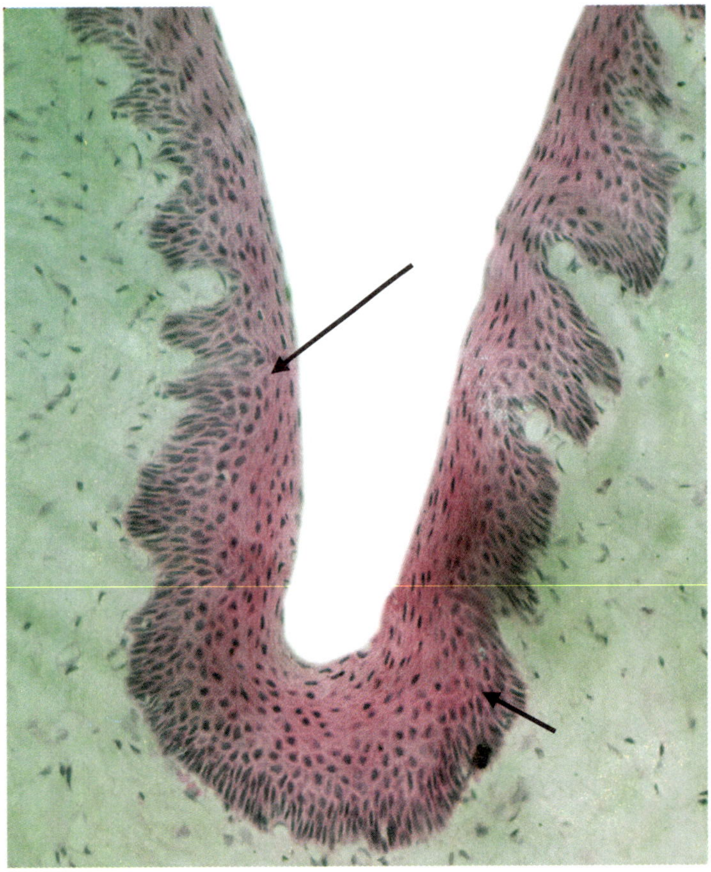

Key Features to Identify the Slide

- Presence of multiple layers of cells
- Basal cell layer is columnar/cuboidal in nature and resting on basement membrane
- Presence of polygonal cell layers with superficial layer of squamous cells

---

Examples

- Oesophagus
- Cornea

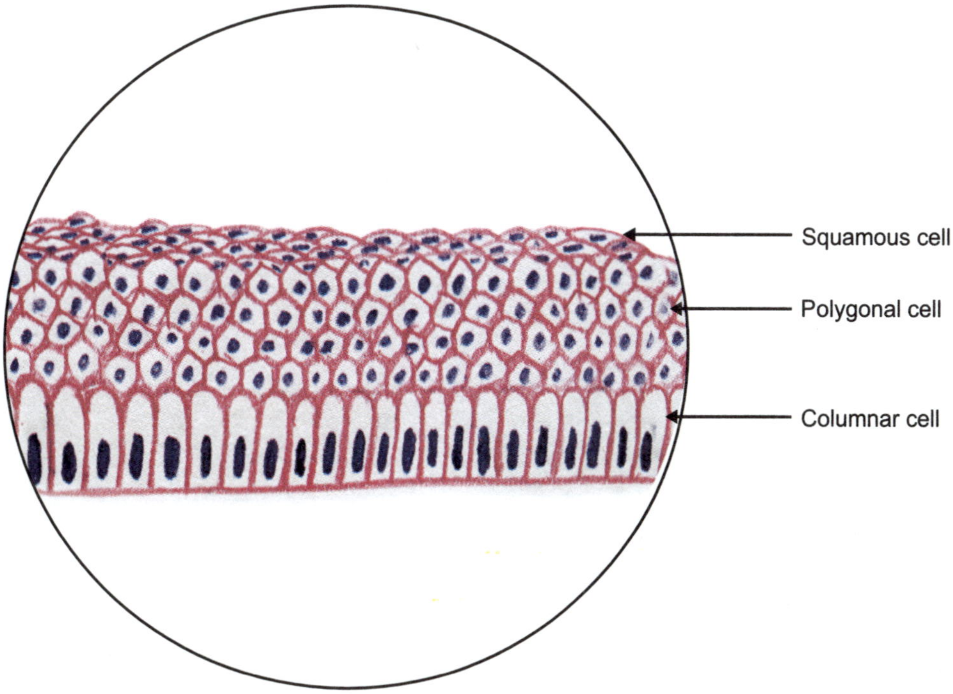
Squamous cell
Polygonal cell
Columnar cell

STRATIFIED SQUAMOUS KERATINIZED EPITHELIUM

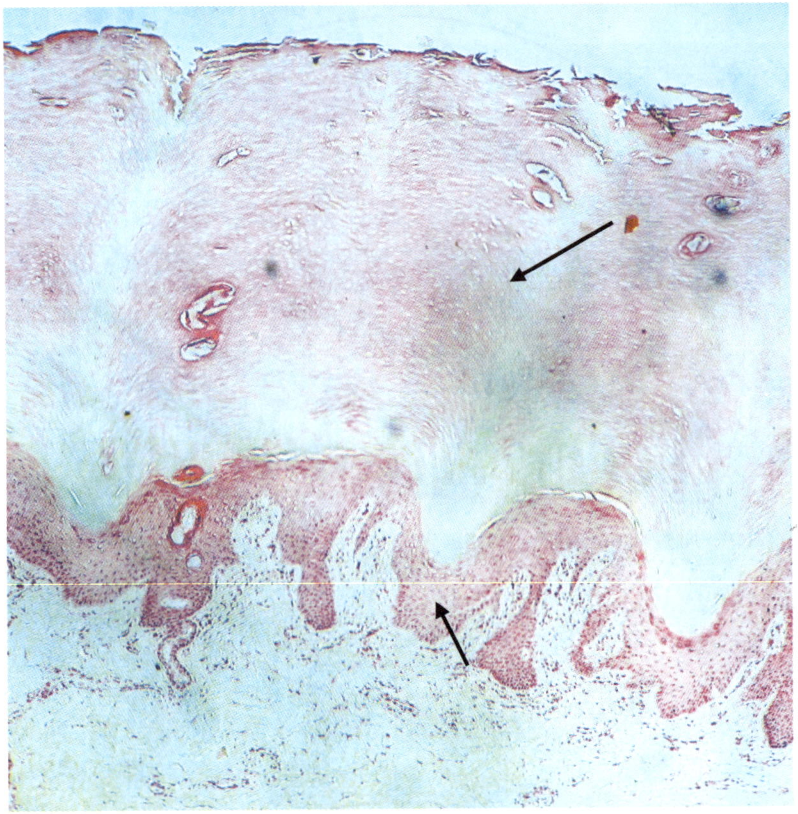

Key Features to Identify the Slide

- Presence of multiple layers of cells
- Basal cell layer is columnar/cuboidal in nature and resting on basement membrane
- Presence of polygonal cell layers with superficial layer of squamous cells
- Presence of well-defined keratin layer on the surface

Examples

- Thick skin
- Thin skin

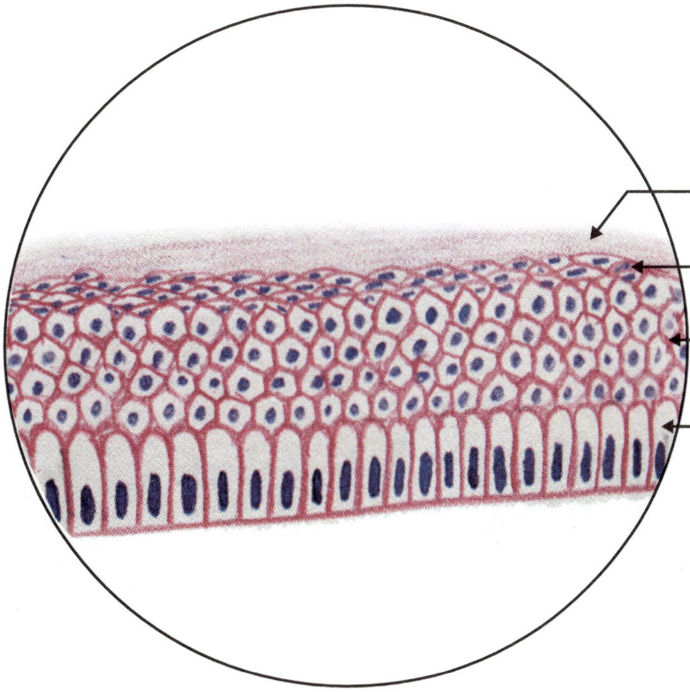
Keratin layer
Squamous cell
Polygonal cell
Columnar cell

TRANSITIONAL EPITHELIUM

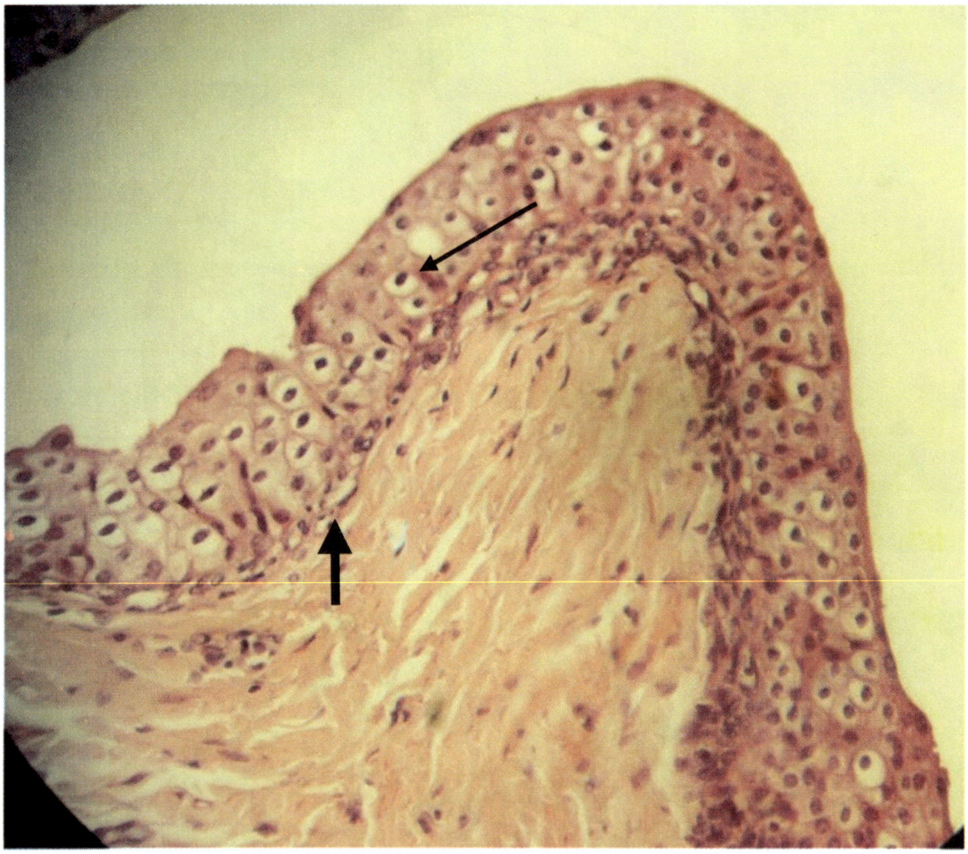

Key Features to Identify the Slide

- Presence of multiple layers of cells
- Basal cell layer is columnar/cuboidal in nature and resting on basement membrane
- Superficial layer made up of umbrella/dome-shaped cells

Examples

- Urinary bladder
- Ureter

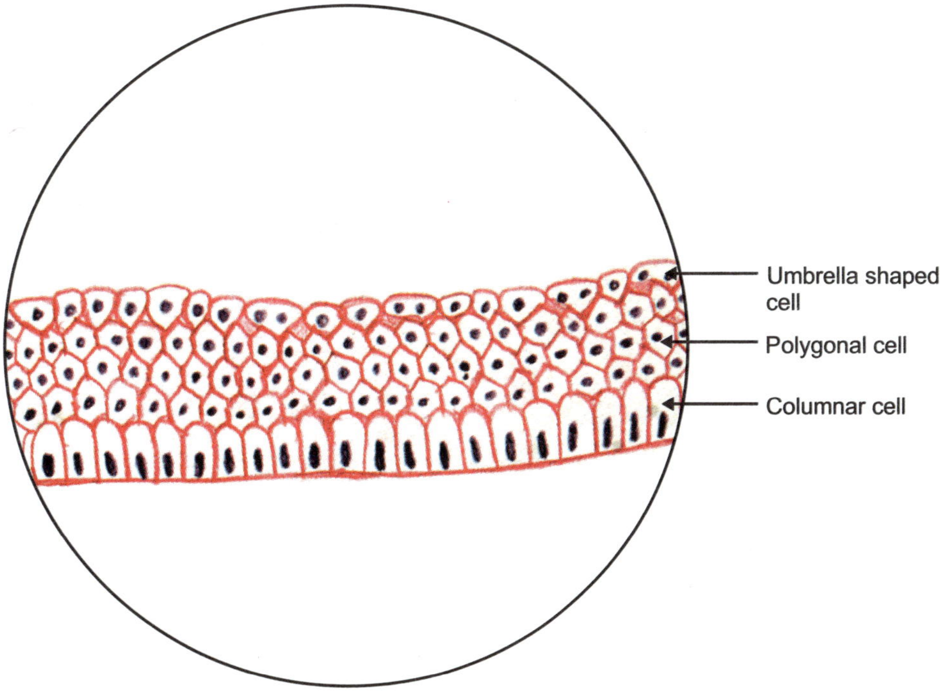
Umbrella shaped cell
Polygonal cell
Columnar cell

QUESTIONS

1. Define epithelium. How does it receive its nutrition? 2M
2. What are the functions of epithelia? 2M
3. What are the surface modifications of epithelial cells? 2M
4. Classify epithelium with suitable diagrams and provide examples for each. 5M
5. What are the types of multicellular glands based on the shape of the secretory units? Provide examples for each type. 2M
6. Classify exocrine glands and provide examples for each. 5M
7. What are the four basic tissues in the body? 2M
8. Describe the junctional complexes. 5M

Figures/Notes

3 Connective Tissue (AN 66.1, 66.2)

- Connective tissue supports and connects other tissues and cells together. It gives metabolic support to cells as the medium for diffusion of nutrients, metabolites and waste products.
- Connective tissue is composed of: 1. cells, and 2. extracellular matrix which consists of fibres and ground substance.
- The variety of connective tissue types in the body reflects differences in composition and amount of the cells, fibres and ground substance.
- General connective tissue which is widespread is classified as loose areolar and dense (irregular and regular) connective tissue.
- Specialised connective tissue includes cartilage and bone.
- Connective tissue consists of (a) collagen fibres—found in most of the supporting tissue, (b) elastic fibres—present in the blood vessels, lung and skin, (c) reticular fibres (type III collagen fibres) —which forms supporting meshwork in liver and lymphoid organs.
- The ground substance present in connective tissue is made up of glycosaminoglycans (dermatan sulphate, keratan sulphate), proteoglycans and glycoproteins.
- Cells of connective tissue are classified as resident and wandering cells.
- Fibroblasts are most common type of supporting cells actively involved in secretion of extracellular matrix in most tissues. Myofibroblasts have contractile function.
- Adipocytes are involved in storage of fat (yellow adipose tissue) and regulation of body temperature in the newborn (brown adipose tissue).

Applied Aspects of Connective Tissue

1. Marfan's syndrome: It is genetic disorder due to abnormal development of elastic fibres affecting large arteries and long bones.
2. Keloid: Scars are formed by fibroblastic activity during tissue repair and it is made up of collagen fibres. Sometimes excessive scar tissue grows beyond the original wound and it is called keloid.

CELLS OF CONNECTIVE TISSUE

Fibroblast

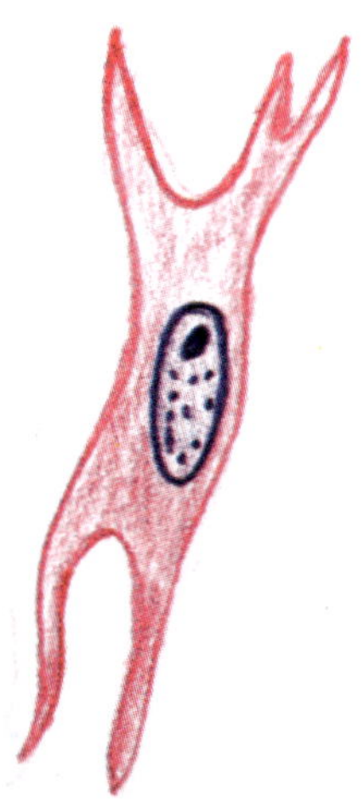

Plasma cell

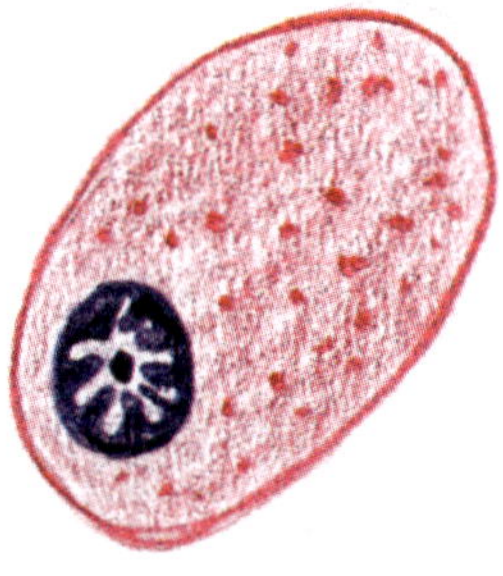

Adipocyte

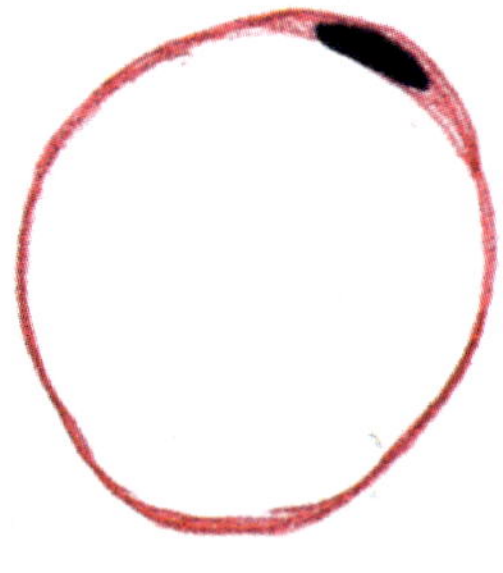

Macrophage

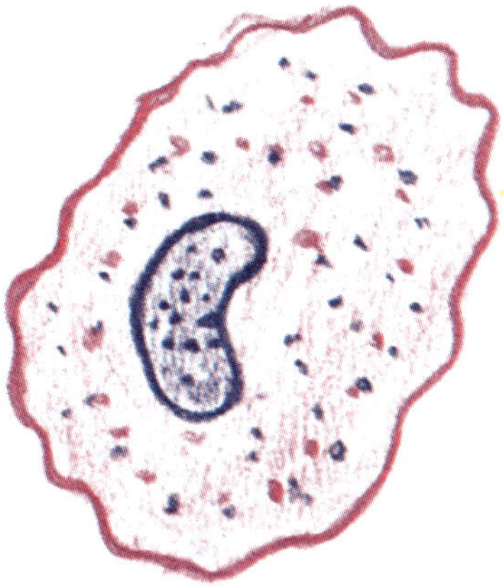

Neutrophil

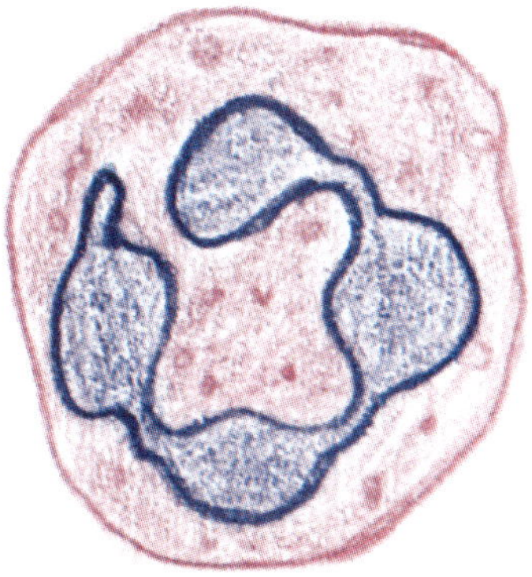

Large lymphocyte

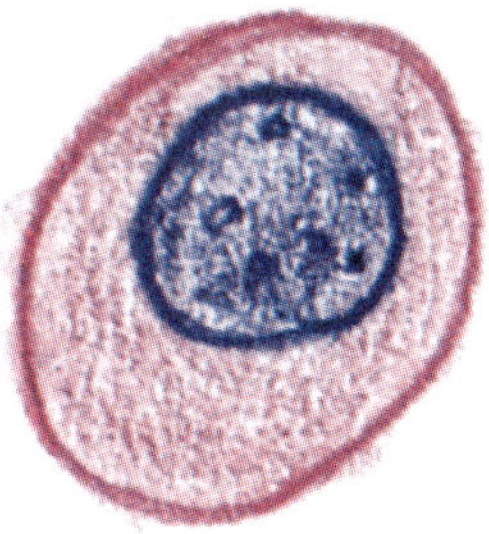

Fibrocyte

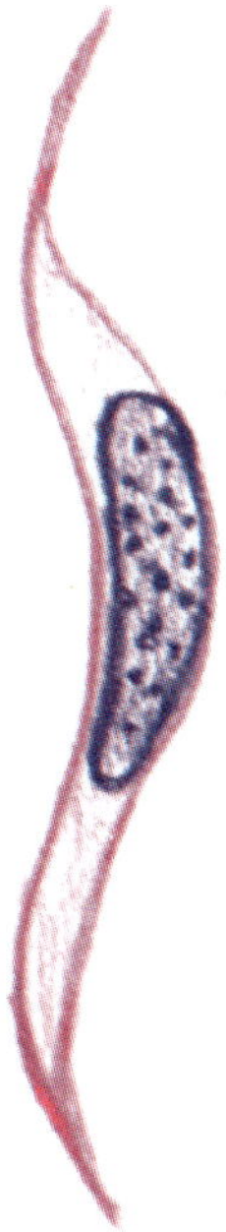

Mast cell

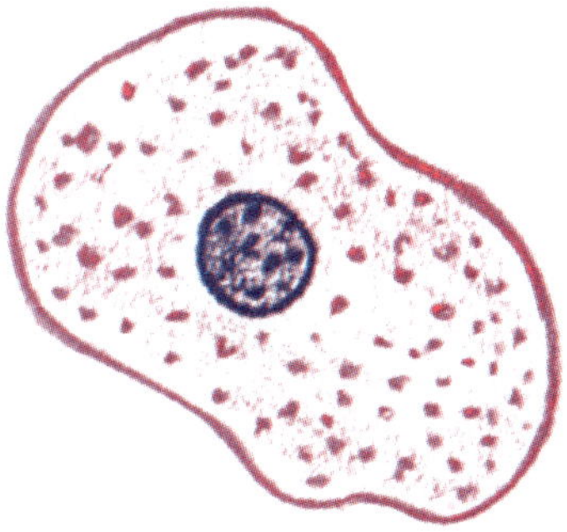

Small lymphocyte

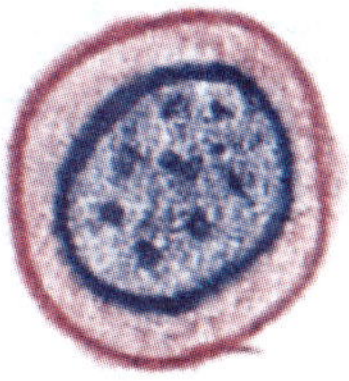

Basophil

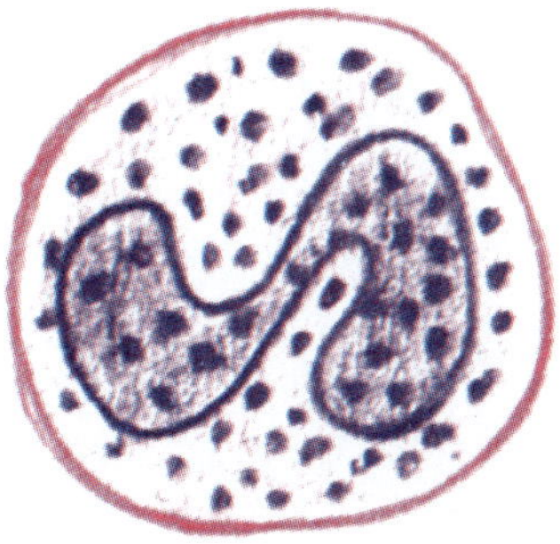

Eosinophil

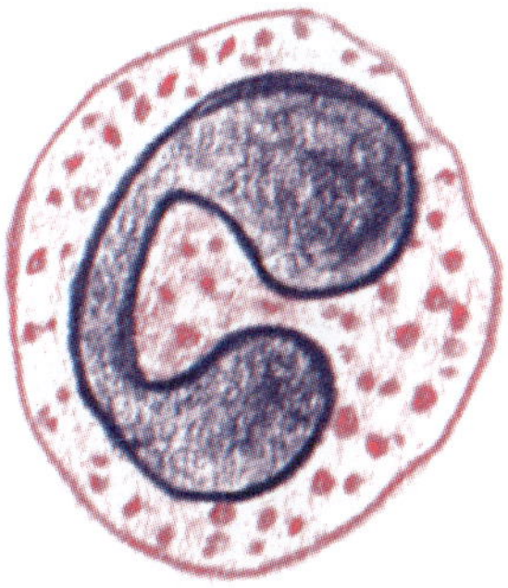

Figures/Notes

Figures/Notes

LOOSE AREOLAR TISSUE

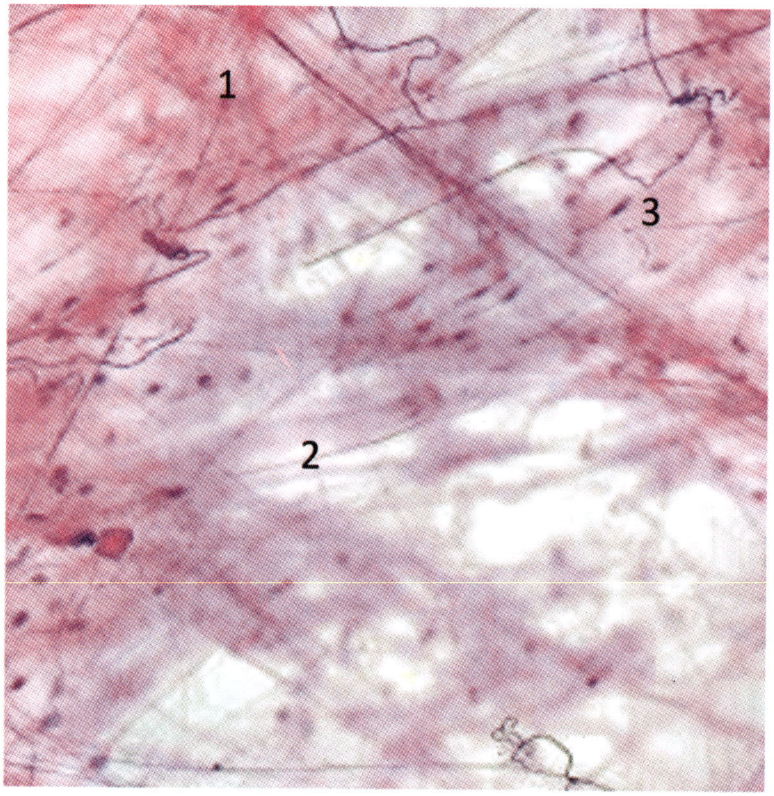

1. Collagen fibres; 2. Elastic fibres; 3. Nuclei of fibroblast

Key Features to Identify the Slide

- Bundles of collagen fibres
- Wavy, branching and anastomosing elastic fibres
- Various connective tissue cells like fibroblast, fibrocytes, mast cells, macrophages, etc.

Examples

- Superficial fascia
- Connective tissue of mesentery

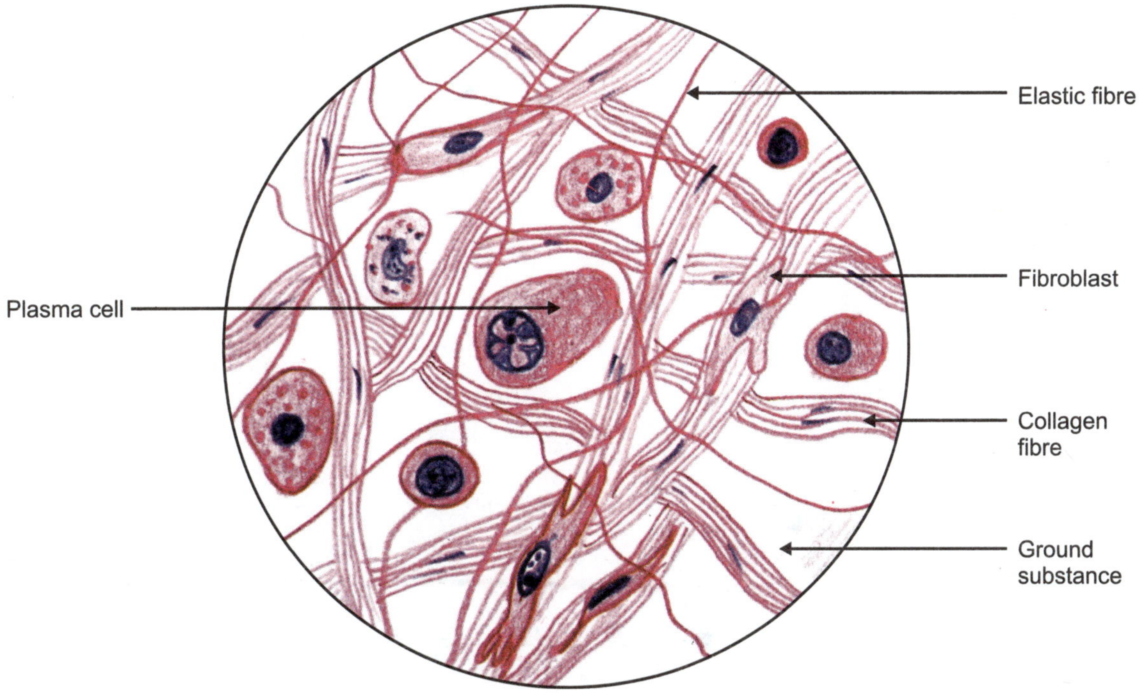
Elastic fibre
Plasma cell
Fibroblast
Collagen fibre
Ground substance

DENSE REGULAR CONNECTIVE TISSUE

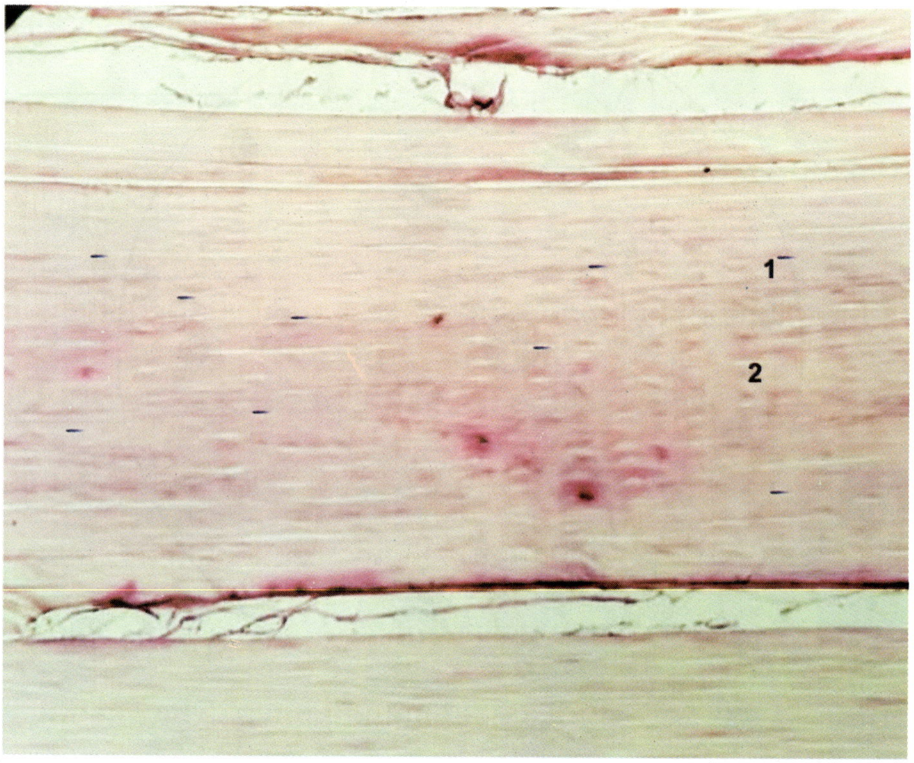

1. Nuclei of fibroblasts; 2. Bundles of collagen fibres

Key Features to Identify the Slide

- Presence of collagen fibres, compactly arranged in parallel bundles
- Nuclei of fibroblasts present in between the bundles of collagen fibres

---

Examples

- Ligaments
- Tendons

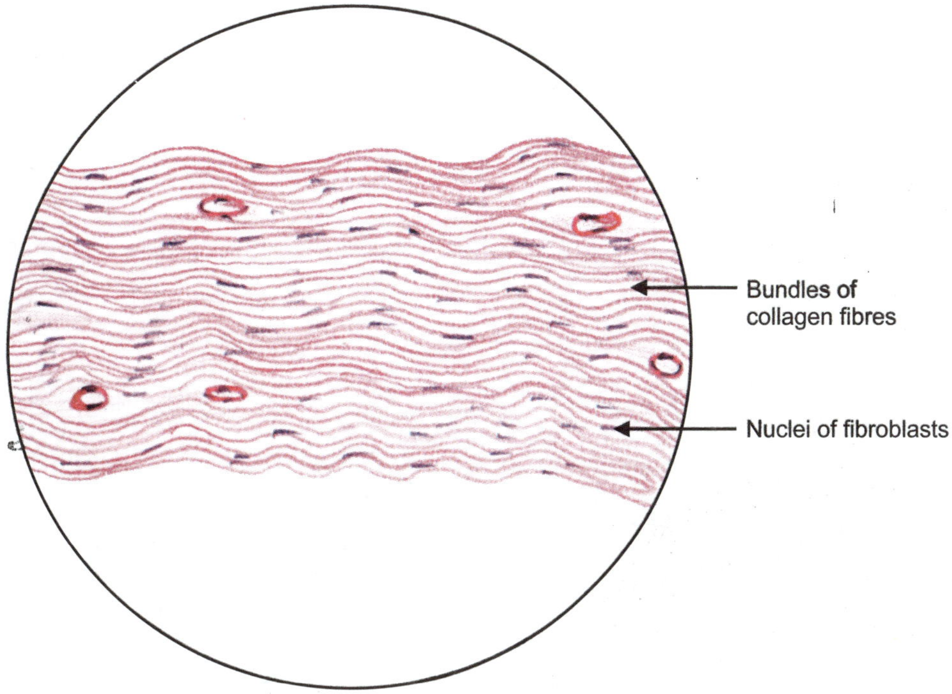
Bundles of
collagen fibres
Nuclei of fibroblasts

DENSE IRREGULAR CONNECTIVE TISSUE

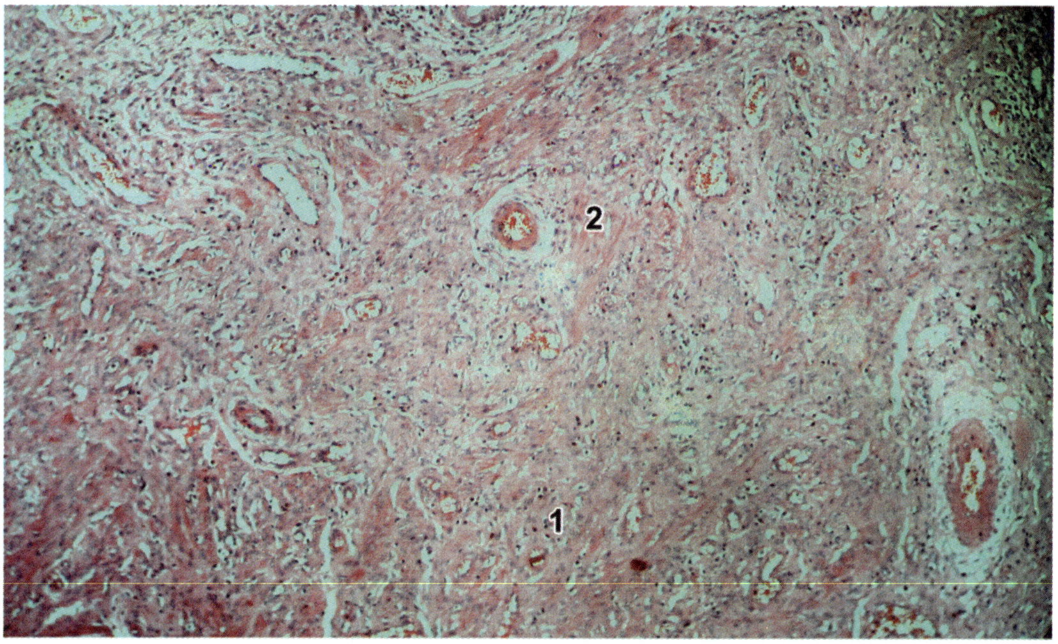

1. Nuclei of fibroblasts; 2. Bundles of collagen fibres

Key Features to Identify the Slide

- Presence of collagen fibres arranged randomly in bundles
- Nuclei of fibroblasts present in between the bundles of collagen fibres

---

Examples

- Dermis of skin
- Dura mater

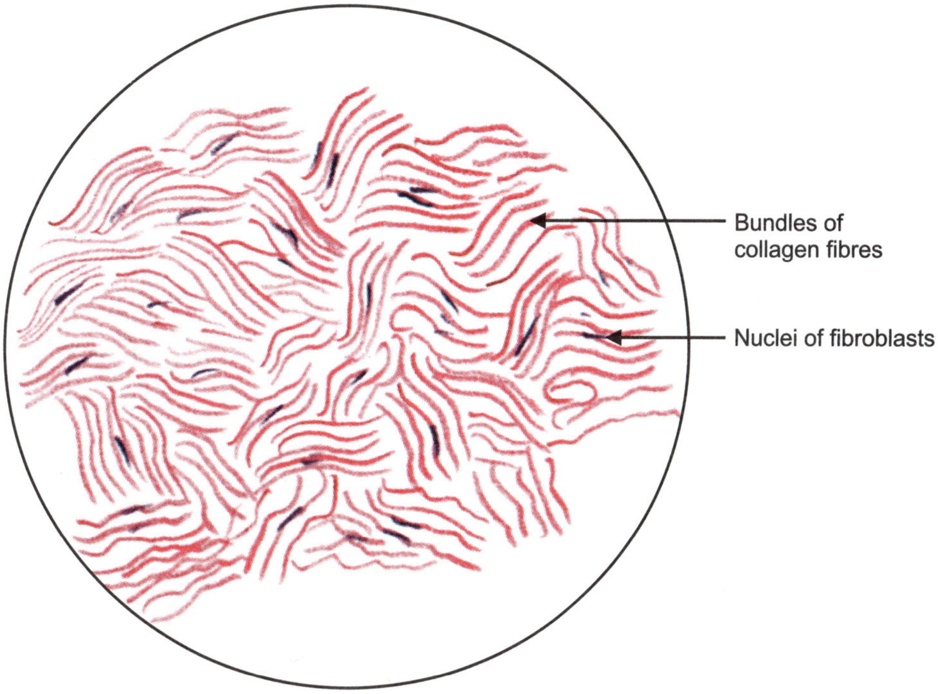
Bundles of
collagen fibres
Nuclei of fibroblasts

ADIPOSE TISSUE

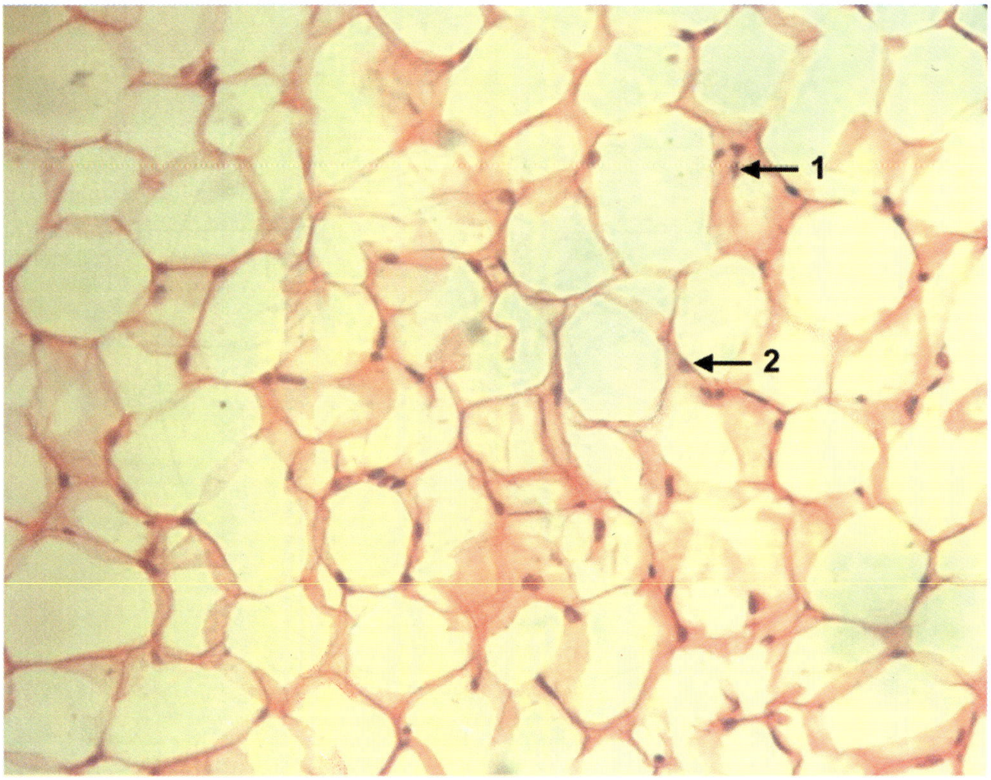

1. Fibroblast; 2. Nuclei of adipose cell

Key Features to Identify the Slide

- Oval/spherical shaped cells
- Vacuolated appearance of cells
- Nucleus pushed to the periphery giving signet ring appearance

---

Examples

- Superficial fascia
- Para-and perirenal fat

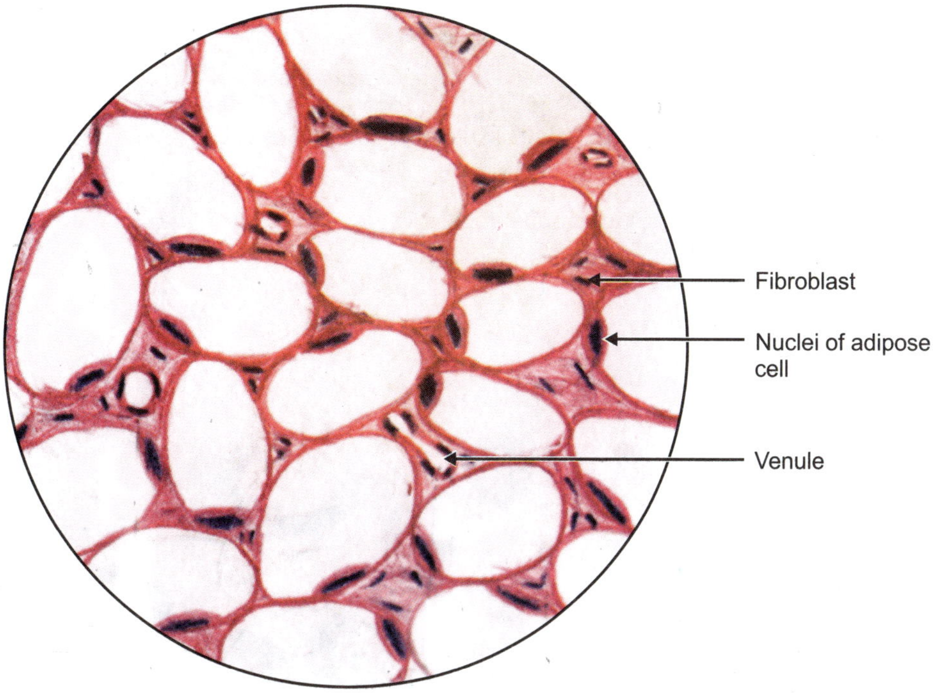
Fibroblast
Nuclei of adipose cell
Venule

QUESTIONS

1. List the components of connective tissue proper. 2M
2. Write a short note on adipose tissue. 5M
3. Describe the structure of the basement membrane. 5M
4. List the functions of fibroblasts. 2M
5. Discuss the different types of cells present in connective tissue. 5M
6. Write the examples of loose connective tissue, dense regular, and irregular connective tissue. 2M
7. Describe the functions of connective tissue. 5M
8. What is the composition of ground substance? 2M
9. Describe the different types of connective tissue. 5M

Figures/Notes

4 Cartilage (AN 71.2)

HYALINE CARTILAGE

1. Perichondrium—covering of the cartilage made up of two layers; outer fibrous and inner cellular (chondrogenic cell layer)
2. Chondrocytes— arranged in the form of isogenous cell nests, they occupy spaces called as lacunae
3. Matrix—transparent and basophilic in nature made up of ground substance and type II collagen fibres. The fibres are not visible in the histological section because of same refractive index as that of ground substance.
   - The territorial matrix (lacunar capsule) surrounding the cell nest is more basophilic, compared to the inter-territorial matrix
   - Growth of the cartilage—cartilage grows by two different methods; interstitial growth and appositional growth
   - Cartilage is avascular, nutrition is provided by surrounding vessels through the process of diffusion

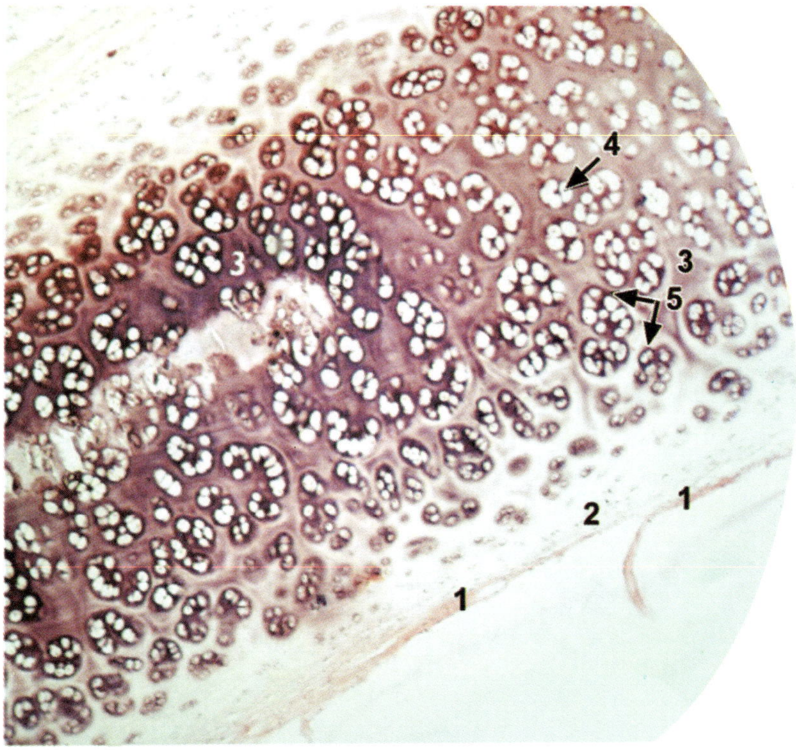

1. Perichondrium (outer fibrous)
2. Perichondrium (inner cellular)
3. Basophilic (homogeneous interterritorial matrix)
4. Lacunae with chondrocytes (cell nests)
5. Territorial matrix

Key Features to Identify the Slide

- Perichondrium covering the surface
- Chondrocytes present in matrix
- Homogeneous basophilic matrix
- Well-defined isogenous cell nests

Examples

– Trachea

– Costal cartilages

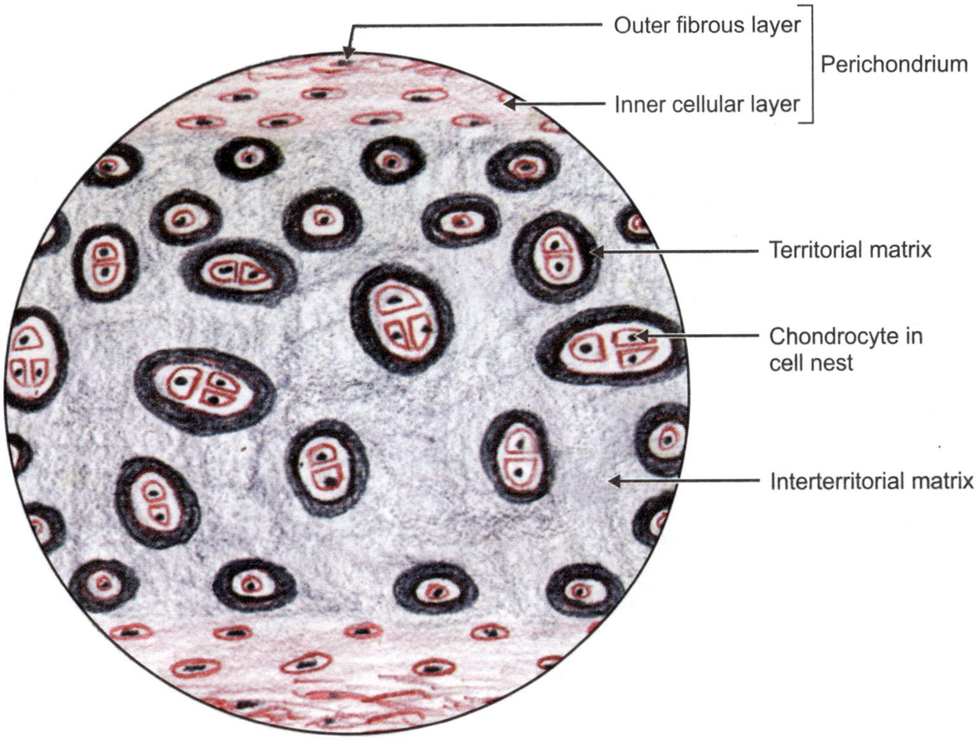
Outer fibrous layer
Inner cellular layer
Perichondrium
Territorial matrix
Chondrocyte in cell nest
Interterritorial matrix

ELASTIC CARTILAGE

1. Perichondrium—covering of the cartilage made up of two layers; outer fibrous and inner cellular (chondrogenic cell layer).
2. Matrix—consists of meshwork of branching and anastomosing elastic fibres. It also contains a few type II collagen fibres.
3. Chondrocytes—present in the lacunae, they are closely packed as the amount of matrix is less when compared to hyaline cartilage.
   - On gross appearance the elastic cartilage appears yellow due to presence of elastic fibres.

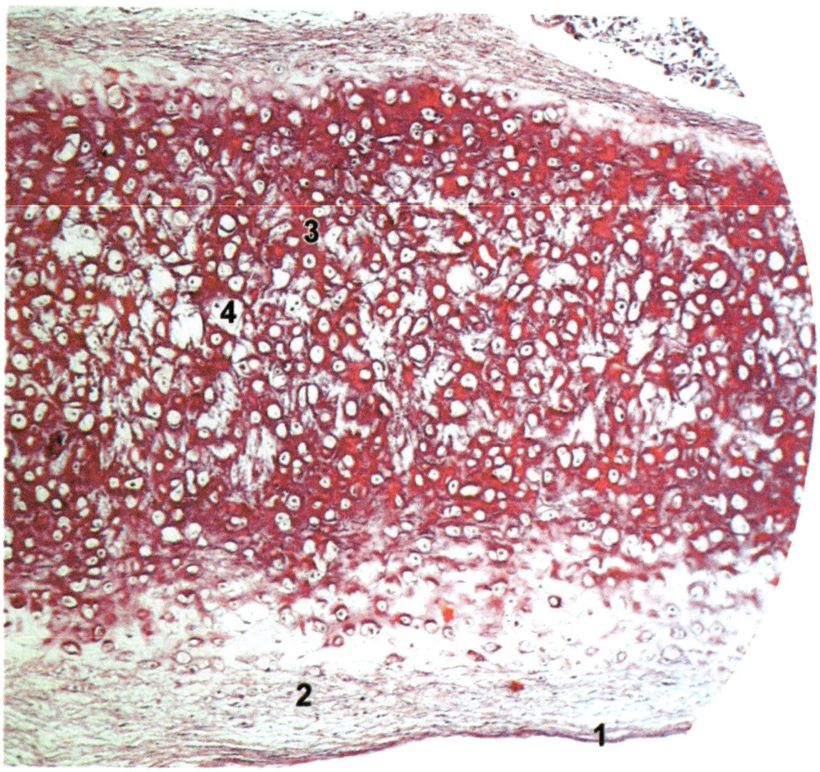

1. Perichondrium (outer fibrous)
2. Perichondrium (inner cellular)
3. Branching and anastomosing elastic fibres in eosinophilic matrix
4. Lacunae with chondrocytes

Key Features to Identify the Slide

- Perichondrium covering the surface
- Matrix rich in elastic fibres
- Cell nests not well defined
- Scanty matrix because of more number of chondrocytes

Examples

- Epiglottis
- Ear pinna

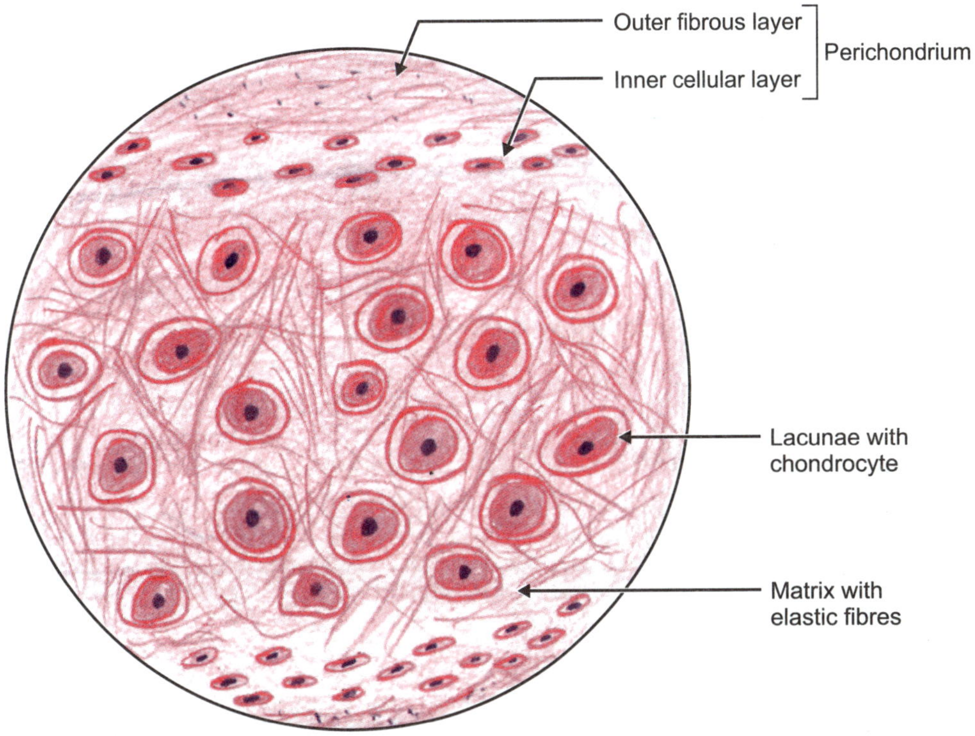
Outer fibrous layer
Inner cellular layer
Perichondrium
Lacunae with chondrocyte
Matrix with elastic fibres

WHITE FIBROCARTILAGE

1. Perichondrium is absent
2. Matrix—consists of bundles of collagen fibres which are oriented in the direction of stress
3. Chondrocytes—arranged in linear rows or scattered singly between the bundles of fibres.

Applied Aspects of Cartilage

1. Osteoarthritis: Inflammation of joints. Articular cartilage undergoes degeneration
2. Chondroma: Benign tumor of cartilage and chondrosarcoma is the malignant tumor.

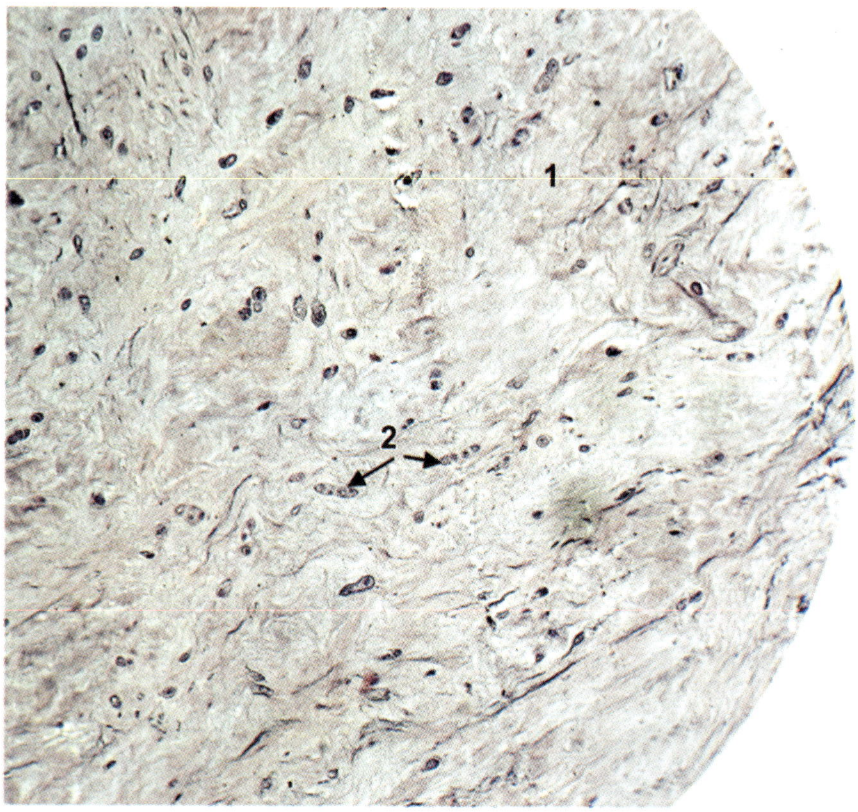

1. Collagen fibres in bundles
2. Chondrocytes (arranged in linear fashion)

Key Features to Identify the Slide

- Perichondrium is absent
- Chondrocytes arranged in linear rows
- Bundles of collagen fibres

Examples

- Intervertebral disc
- Menisci of knee joint

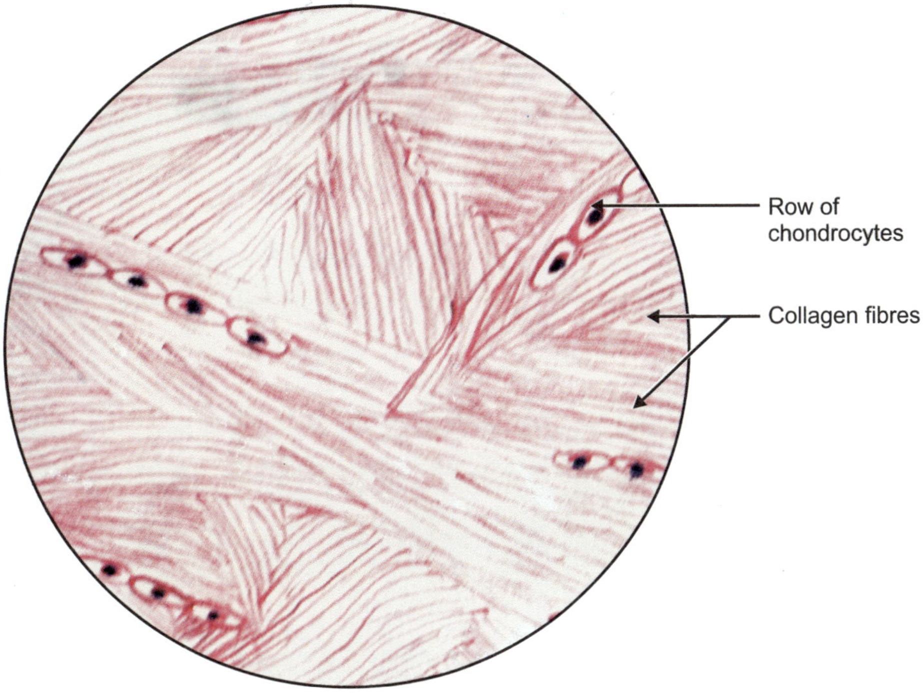
Row of chondrocytes
Collagen fibres

QUESTIONS

1. Define perichondrium. 2M
2. Elaborate on the microscopic structure of various types of cartilage with examples. 5M
3. Enumerate the functions of cartilage. 2M
4. Explore the rationale behind the dark appearance of the territorial matrix in hyaline cartilage. 2M
5. Microanatomy of hyaline cartilage. 5M
6. Microanatomy of elastic cartilage. 5M
7. Microanatomy of white fibrocartilage. 5M

Figures/Notes

COMPACT BONE: TRANSVERSE SECTION (TS)

Periosteum—outer covering of the bone consisting of two layers outer fibrous and inner cellular layer

Haversian system/osteon—it is a structural unit of compact bone; it consists of a single central canal (Haversian canal) with surrounding 4–15 concentric lamellae.

- Canal contains connective tissue, capillaries, nerves and lymphatics
- Between the lamellae there are spaces called lacunae that contains osteocytes
- Lamellae—based on the location lamellae are classified as: 1. Inner circumferential lamellae (present around the marrow cavity), 2. Outer circumferential—present beneath the periosteum, 3. Interstitial—present in between the osteons.

Types of cells present in the bone: Osteoblasts, osteocytes, osteoclasts and osteoprogenitor cells.

Bone matrix—consists of type 1 collagen fibres and ground substance with inorganic salts of calcium and phosphate.

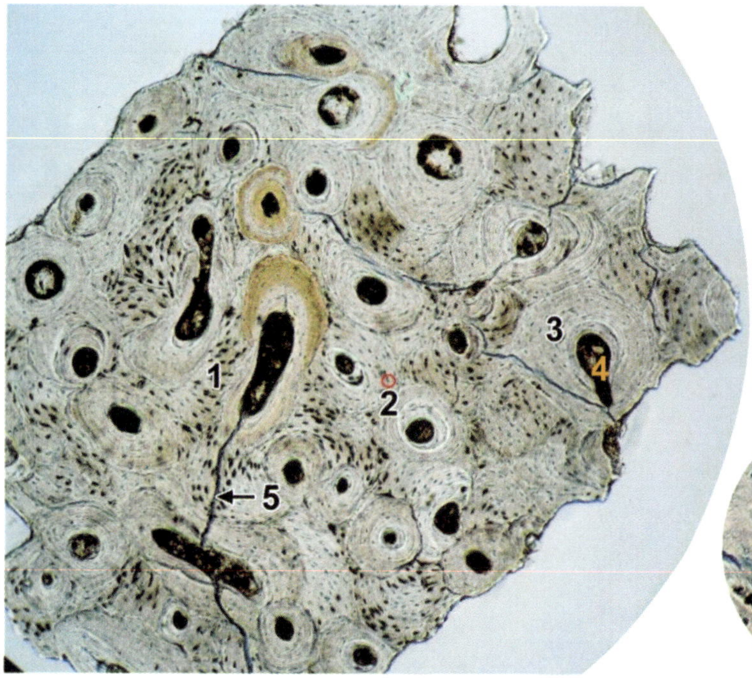

1. Interstitial lamellae
2. Osteocytes within the lacunae
3. Lamellae
4. Central (Haversian) canal
5. Volkmann's canal

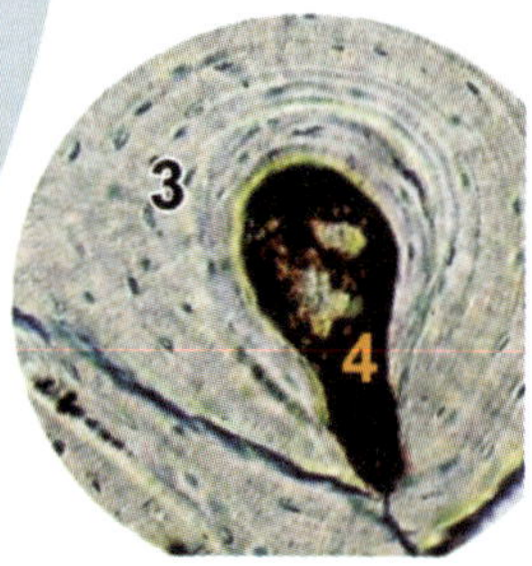

Osteon

Key Features to Identify the Slide

- Haversian system (osteon) is seen
- Osteocytes in lacunae
- Different types of lamellae
- Volkmann's canal (horizontally placed)
- Periosteum—outermost layer

Examples

- Diaphysis/shaft of long bones
- Outer and inner table of skull

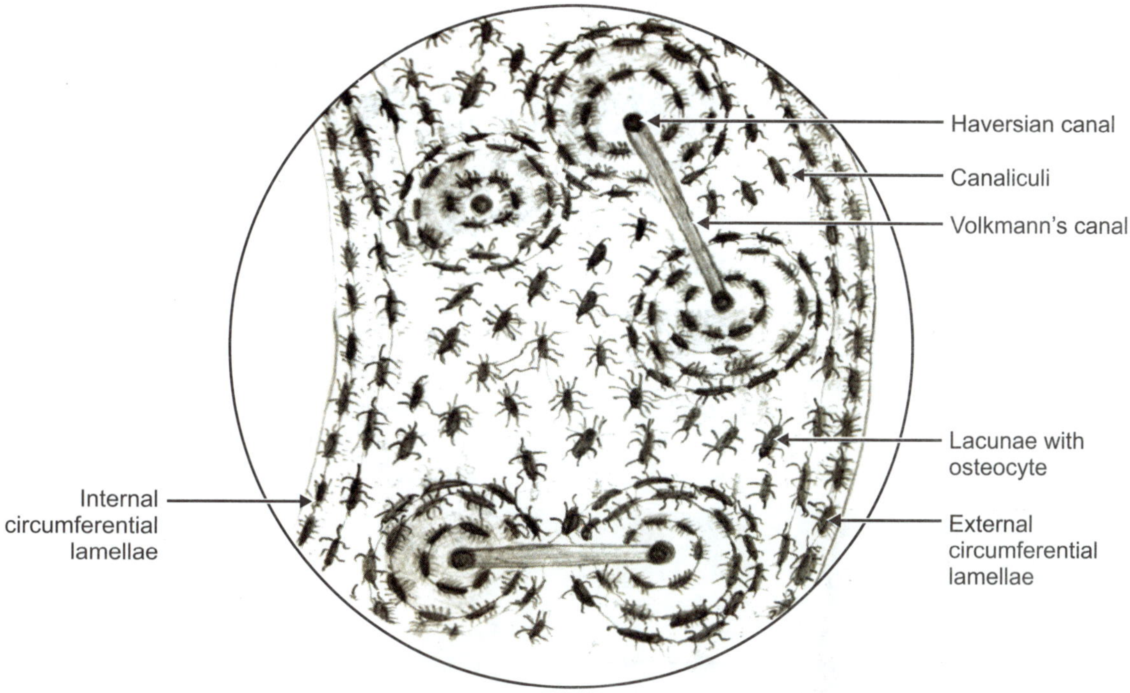
Haversian canal
Canaliculi
Volkmann's canal
Lacunae with osteocyte
External circumferential lamellae
Internal circumferential lamellae

COMPACT BONE: LONGITUDINAL SECTION (LS)

Periosteum:

(a) Outer fibrous layer: Made up of collagen fibres, these fibres binding the periosteum to the bone are called Sharpey's fibres

(b) Inner cellular layer: It is the osteogenic layer which can differentiate into osteoblast.

Volkmann's canal—Haversian canal of one osteon is connected with the other osteon by Volkmann's canal. They are horizontally or obliquely placed in relation to the long axis of the bone. They also connect with periosteum and endosteum.

Lamellae—are placed parallel to each other along the long axis of the bone.

- In between the lamellae osteocytes along with their cytoplasmic processes are present in spaces called lacunae with their canaliculi.

Applied Aspects of Bone

1. Osteoporosis: Reduction in density of bone due to increased resorption leading to frequent fractures.
2. Rickets: Vitamin D deficiency leads to inadequate mineralization of bone which causes bowing of long bones.

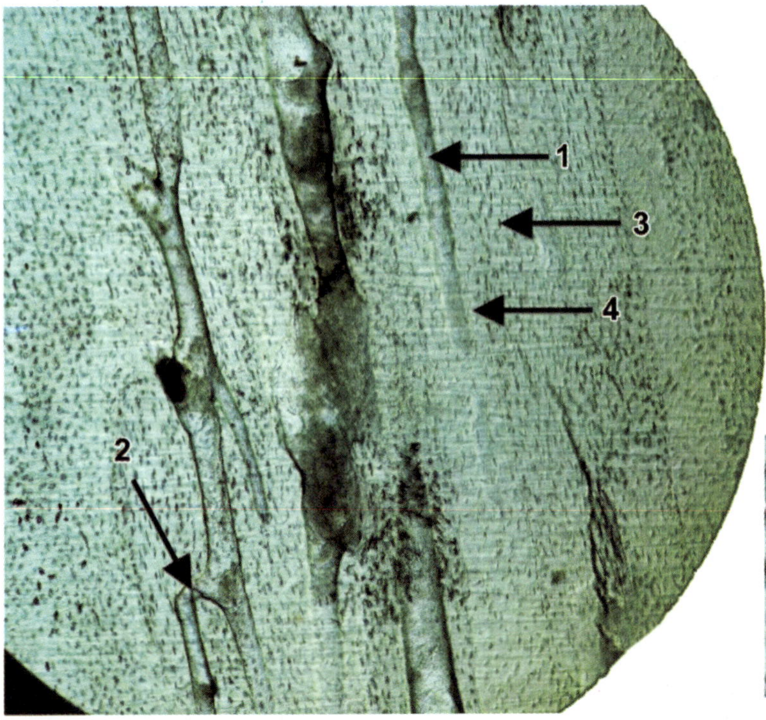

1. Central (Haversian) canal
2. Perforating (Volkmann's) canal
3. Lacunae
4. Lamellae

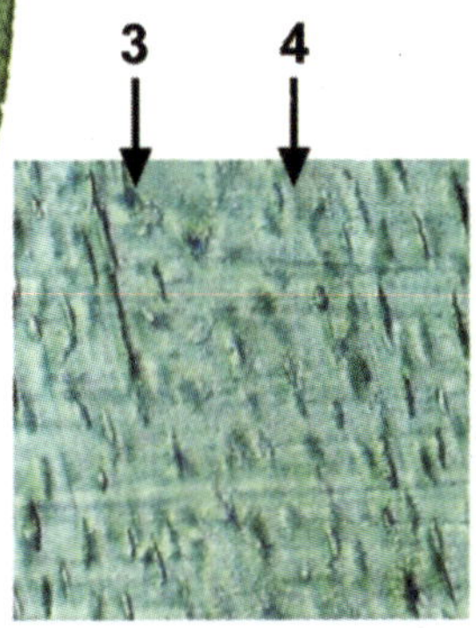

Key Features to Identify the Slide

- Haversian canal—vertically placed
- Volkmann's canal—horizontally placed
- Osteocytes in lacunae
- Presence of lamellae

Examples

- Diaphysis/shaft of long bones
- Outer and inner table of skull

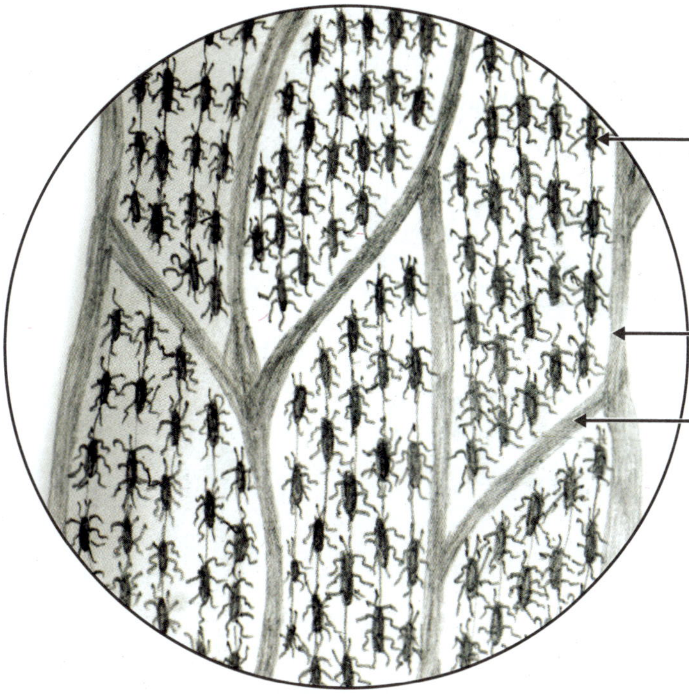
Lacunae with
osteocyte
Haversian canal
Volkmann's
canal

QUESTIONS

1. Define and describe the structure of an osteon. 5M
2. Enumerate the types of bone cells and their respective locations and functions. 5M
3. Name the components comprising the bone matrix. 2M
4. Name the layers of perichondrium and their functions. 2M
5. Name the bone cells involved in fracture healing. 2M
6. Define periosteum and endosteum. 2M
7. Write in detail the processes of intramembranous and endochondral ossification. 5M
8. Define spongy bone with an example. 2M
9. Define Howship's lacuna. 2M
10. Explain the significance of Sharpey's fibres. 2M
11. Specify the organic and inorganic constituents of the bone matrix. 2M

Figures/Notes

6 Muscle Tissue (AN 67.1, 67.2)

SKELETAL MUSCLE: TRANSVERSE SECTION (TS)

Epimysium: Covering the entire muscle. Made up of loose connective tissue rich in collagen and elastic fibres.

Perimysium: Covering each muscle fasciculus/bundle

- Is made up of thick bundle of collagen fibres

Endomysium: Covering the individual muscle fibre

- Made up of thin layer of reticular fibres

Functions of connective tissue sheath: They transmit the force of contraction to the neighbouring fibres.

- They provide passage for the blood vessels and nerves

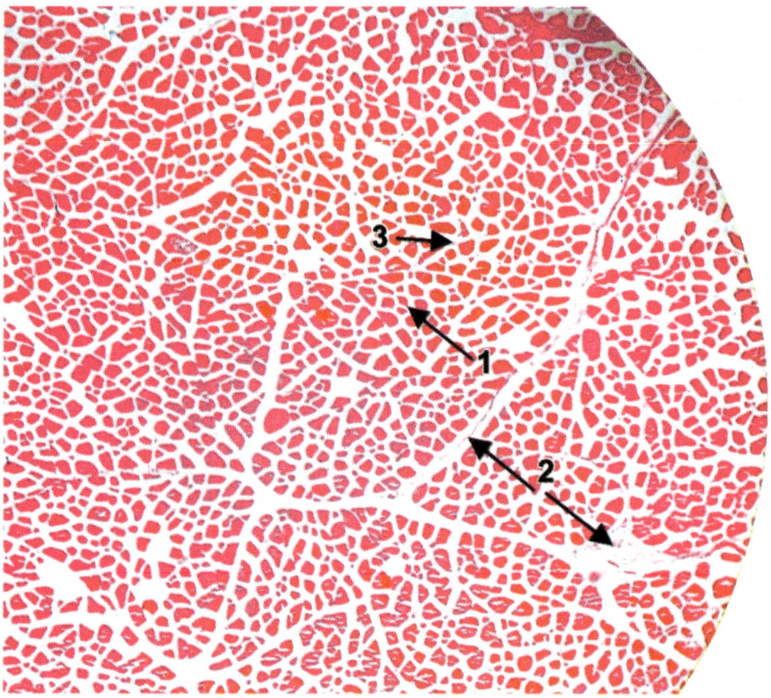

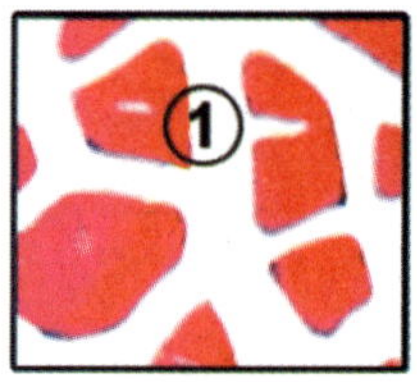

1. Transverse section of muscle fibre with peripheral nucleus
2. Perimysium
3. Endomysium

Key Features to Identify the Slide

Connective tissue sheaths in the form of:

- Epimysium—covering entire skeletal muscle
- Perimysium—covering the muscle fascicles
- Endomysium—covering individual muscle cell
- Peripherally placed nucleus

Examples

- Deltoid
- Gluteus maximus

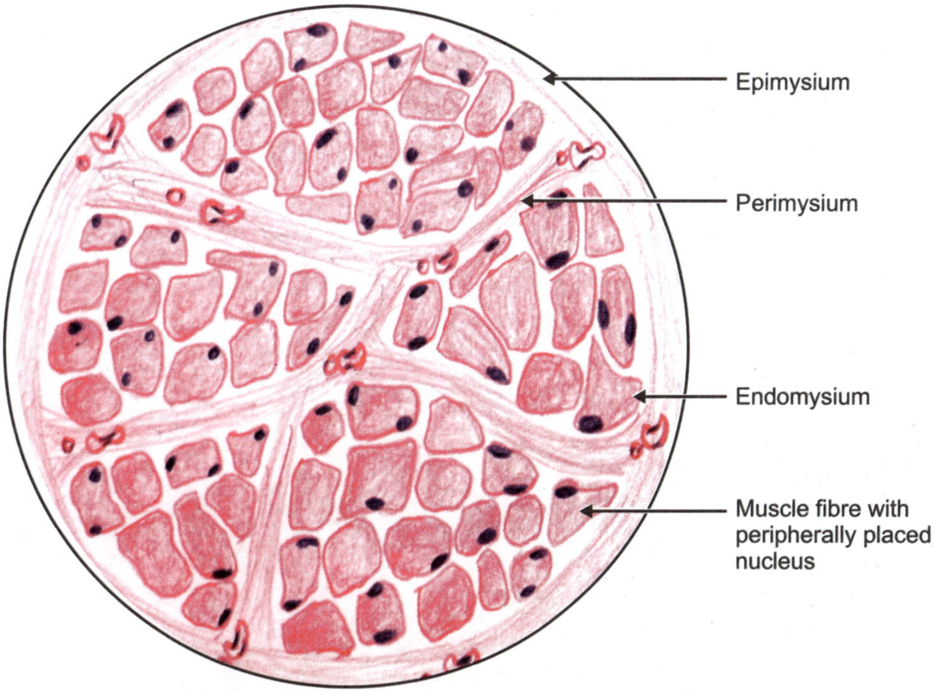
Epimysium
Perimysium
Endomysium
Muscle fibre with peripherally placed nucleus

SKELETAL MUSCLE: LONGITUDINAL SECTION (LS)

Muscle fibre: Each muscle fibre exhibits dark and light bands (striations).

- It is multinucleated and nucleus is peripherally placed beneath the cell membrane because cytoplasm or the sarcoplasm is occupied by contractile filaments actin and myosin.

Sarcomere: Contractile unit of the muscle. It is this segment of myofibril between two adjacent z-lines.

Muscle triad: The sarcoplasmic reticulum forms terminal cisternae on either side of T-tubules at each A and I band junction.

- It plays an important role in muscle contraction.
- Contraction is voluntary in nature being innervated by somatic nerve fibres.

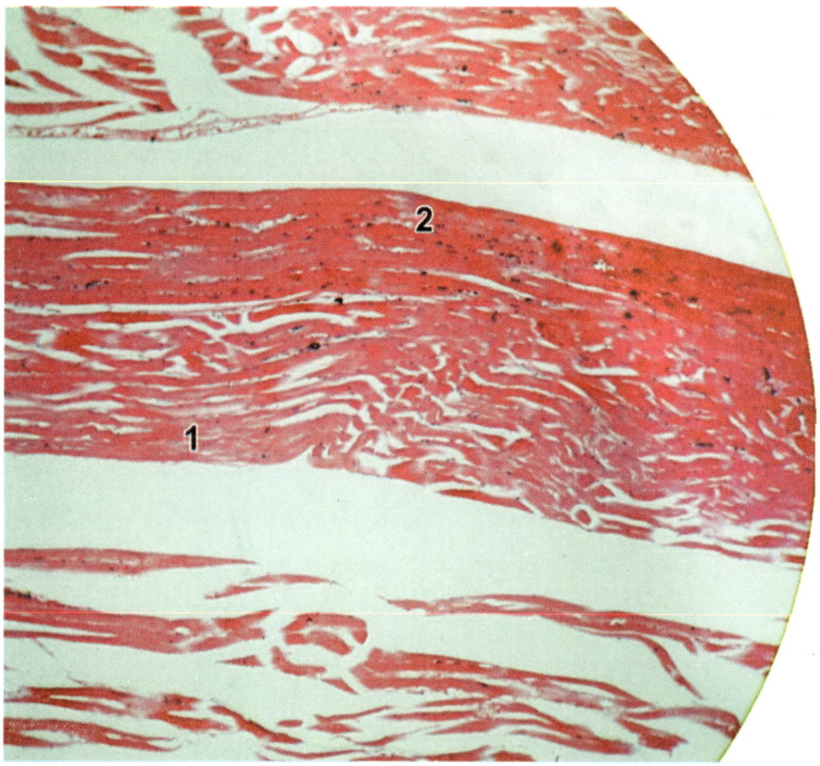

1. Long cylindrical and unbranched muscle fibres
2. Peripheral nucleus (multinucleated arranged in chains)

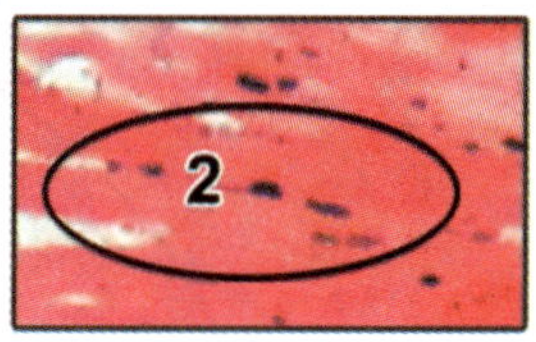

Key Features to Identify the Slide

- Parallel arrangement of cylindrical muscle fibres
- No branching of muscle fibres
- Multiple nuclei at periphery
- Striations are seen

Examples

- Deltoid
- Gluteus maximus

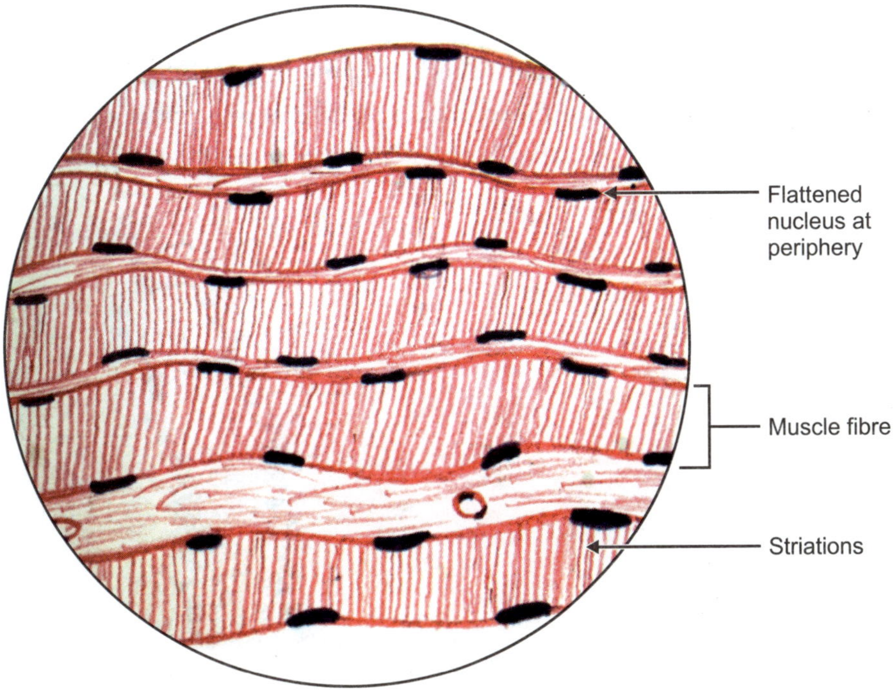
Flattened nucleus at periphery
Muscle fibre
Striations

CARDIAC MUSCLE

Muscle fibre: Cardiac muscle fibre also exhibit cross striations like skeletal muscle but not so prominent as they have few myofibrils.

Intercalated disc: These are specialised junction between two cardiac myocytes.

- They have a staircase like arrangement because of the presence of gap junctions and **desmosomes**.
- This arrangement will facilitate the contraction of cardiac muscle as a single **unit (syncytium)**.
- Contraction is involuntary in nature being innervated by autonomic **nerve fibres**.

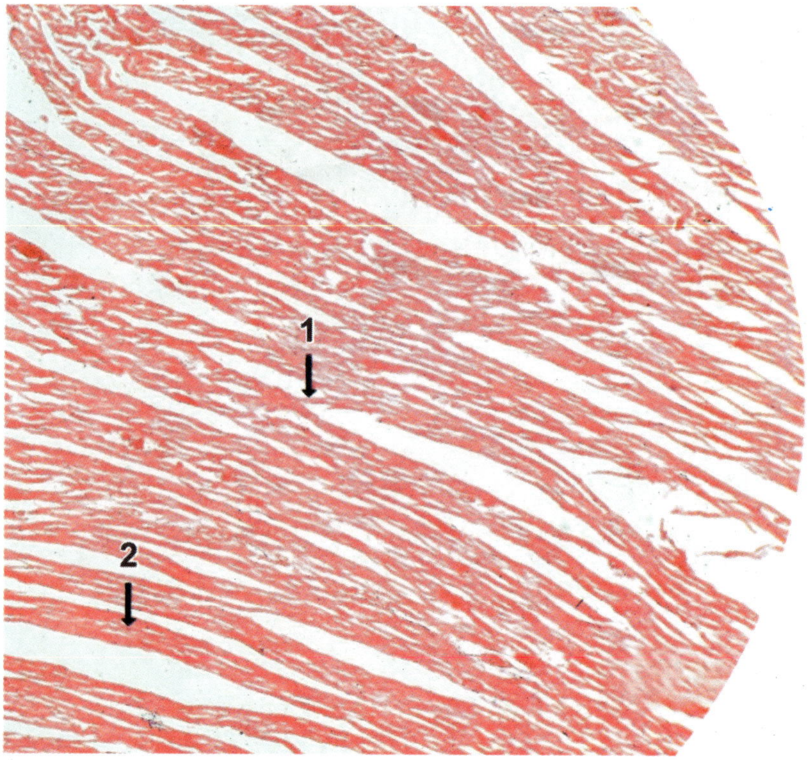

1. Branching and anastomosing muscle fibres
2. Central nucleus

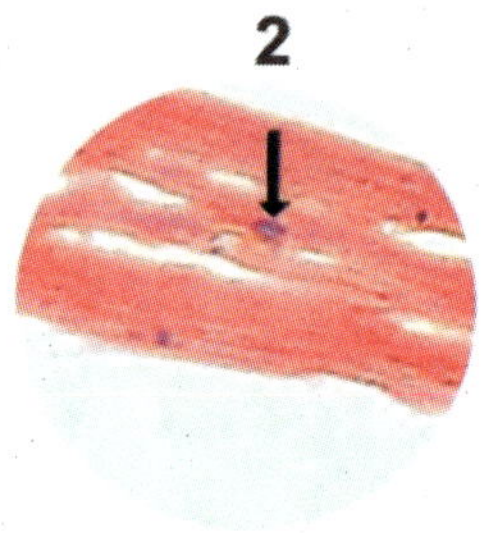

Key Features to Identify the Slide

- Short cylindrical muscle fibres
- Branching and anastomosing pattern of muscle fibres
- Single oval nucleus at centre
- Intercalated discs are present

Example

– Myocardium of heart

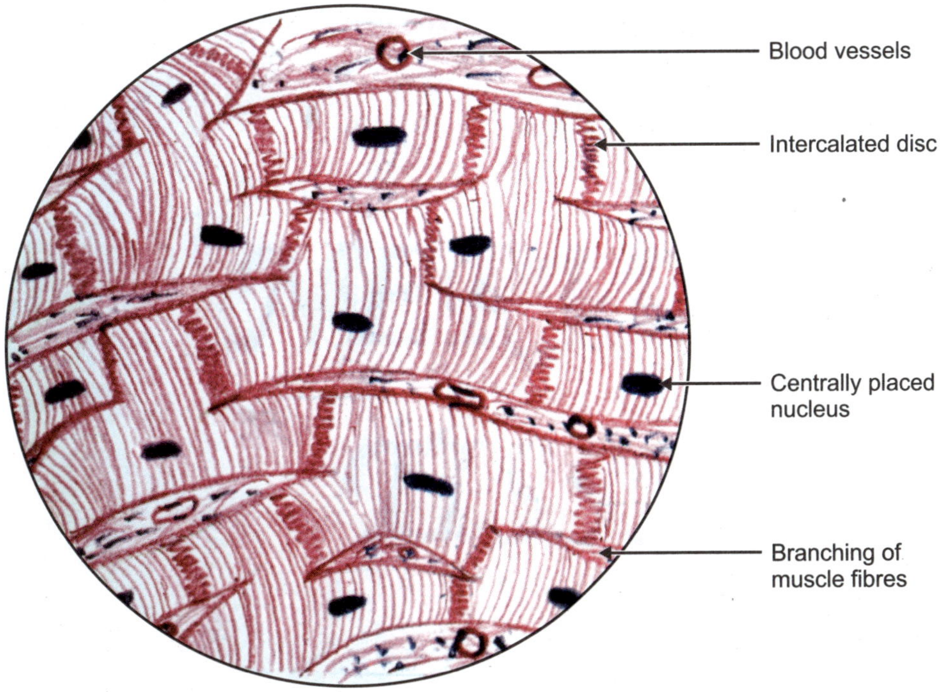
Blood vessels
Intercalated disc
Centrally placed nucleus
Branching of muscle fibres

SMOOTH MUSCLE

Muscle fibre: They are arranged in the form of a well-defined circular and longitudinal layers.

- They contain actin and myosin filaments but they do not exhibit striations as they are not arranged in an orderly manner
- Smooth muscle contains intermediate filaments which helps in shortening of muscle cell during contraction (cork screw pattern)
- Involuntary being supplied by autonomic nerve fibres.

They are classified into two categories based on innervation as single unit and multi-unit smooth muscle.

Applied Aspects of Muscle Tissue

1. Hypertrophy—enlargement of individual muscle fibres in response to stress.
2. Hyperplasia—increase in number of muscle fibres as in smooth muscles of uterus.

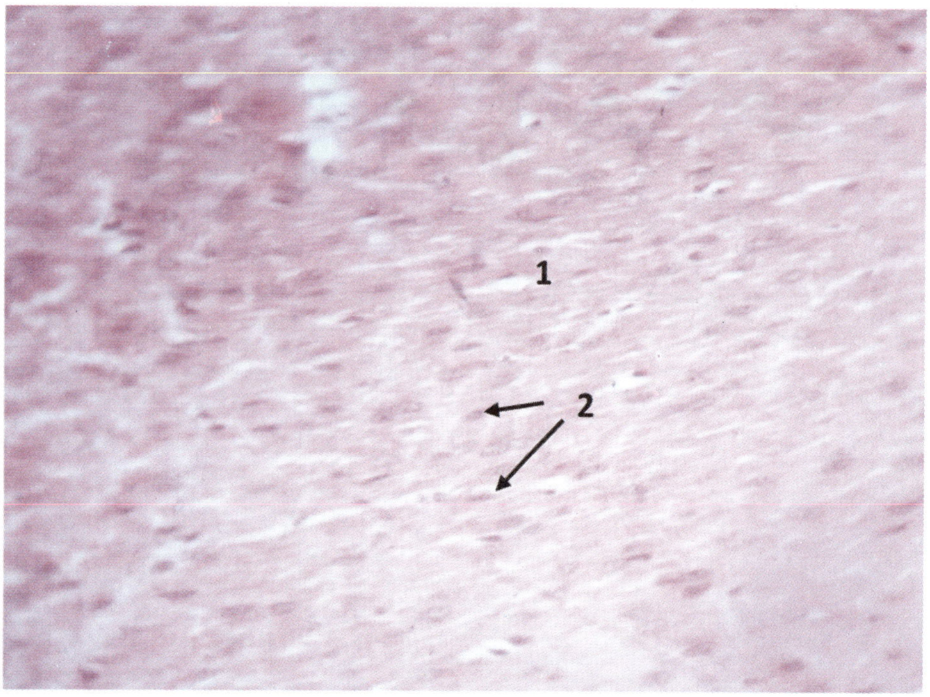

1. Muscle fibres
2. Nuclei of muscle fibres

Key Features to Identify the Slide

- Spindle-shaped muscle fibres
- Fibres arranged in well-defined layers
- Elongated nucleus situated in the centre

Examples

- Urinary bladder
- Stomach

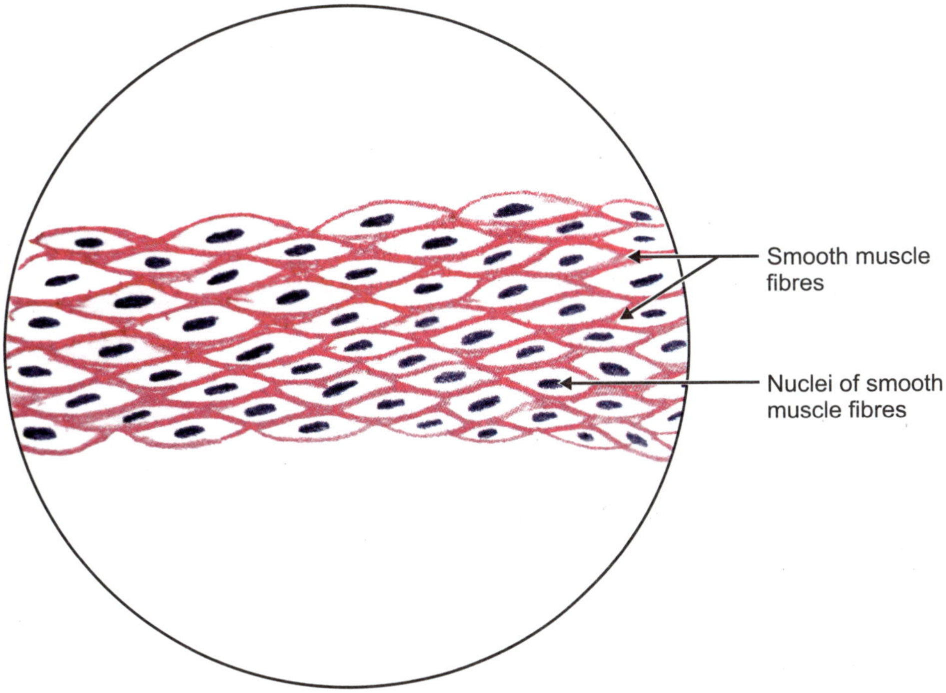
Smooth muscle fibres
Nuclei of smooth muscle fibres

QUESTIONS

1. Elaborate on the microscopic characteristics of skeletal muscle and elucidate the factors responsible for the development of striations in skeletal muscle. 5M
2. Discuss the microscopic features observed in transverse section of skeletal muscle tissue. 5M
3. Define the concept of triad in the context of skeletal muscle. 2M
4. Microscopic structure of cardiac muscle. 5M
5. What is intercalated disc. 2M
6. Examine the variations between smooth and skeletal muscles in terms of their structural and functional characteristics. 5M

Figures/Notes

7 Nervous Tissue (AN 68.1,68.2,68.3)

Peripheral Nerve: Transverse Section (TS)

Epineurium: It surrounds entire nerve and is made up of connective tissue.

Perineurium: It surrounds bundles (fasciculi) of nerve fibres.

- It is a connective tissue sheath made up of two to three layers of flattened cells and covered externally by basal lamina.

Endoneurium: It surrounds individual nerve fibre and made up of thin layer of connective tissue.

- These connective tissue sheaths carry blood vessels which supply the nerve fibres.

Myelin sheath: Surrounding each axon takes up of osmium stain and appears dark in colour.

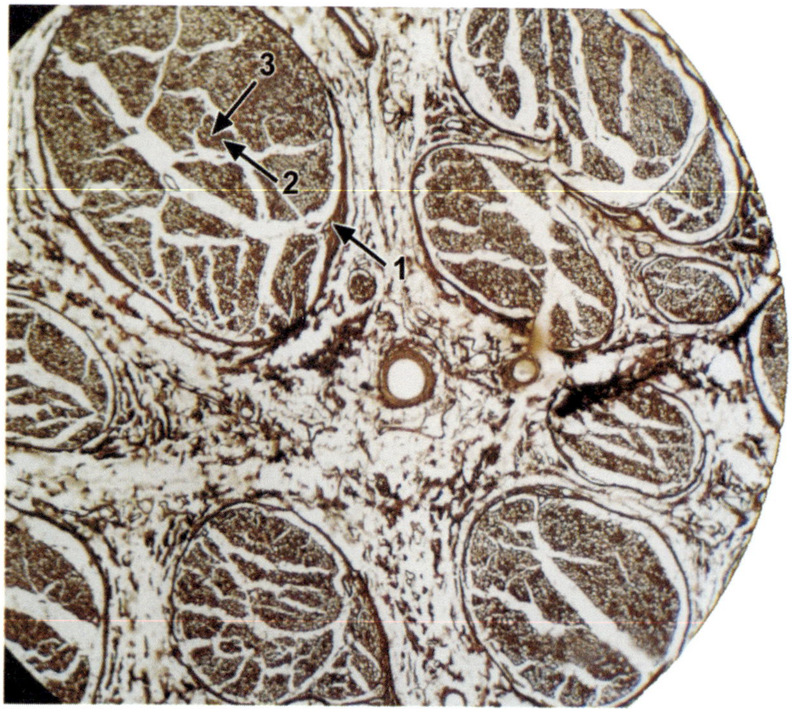

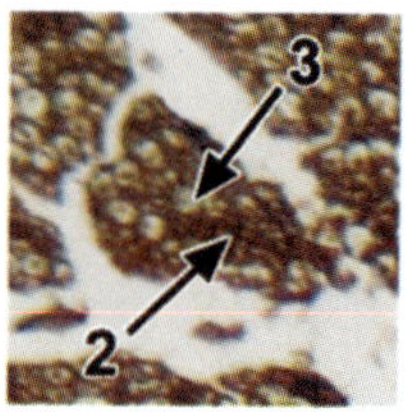

1. Perineurium
2. Axon surrounded by endoneurium
3. Myelin sheath around the axon

Key Features to Identify the Slide

[Osmic acid stain]

- Transversely cut nerve fibres arranged in bundles
- Epineurium covering the whole nerve
- Perineurium covering the bundles of nerve fibres
- Endoneurium covering each nerve fibre

Examples

- Radial nerve
- Sciatic nerve

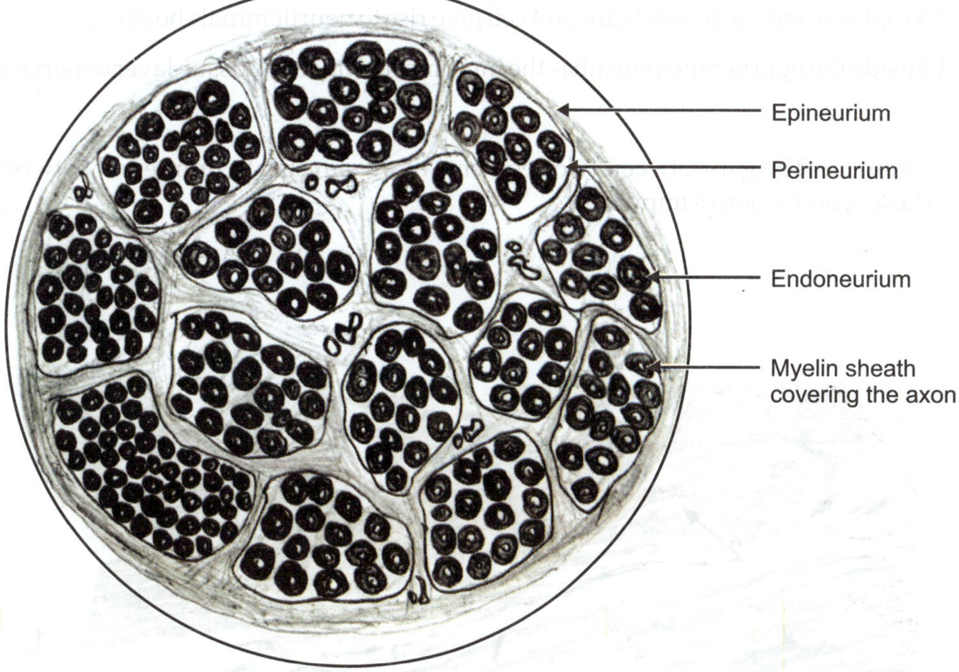
Epineurium
Perineurium
Endoneurium
Myelin sheath covering the axon

Peripheral Nerve: Longitudinal Section (LS)

Each axon/peripheral nerve has axolemma (cell membrane) which surrounds the cytoplasm (axoplasm).

- Outside axolemma there is presence of myelin sheath which is synthesized by Schwann cell.
- Cytoplasm and nucleus of Schwann cell give rise to neurilemmal sheath.
- Outside the neurilemmal sheath is the innermost connective tissue layer of nerve that is endoneurium.

Node of Ranvier: The gap between two segments of myelin sheath or interval between two Schwann cells which helps in faster conduction of impulses.

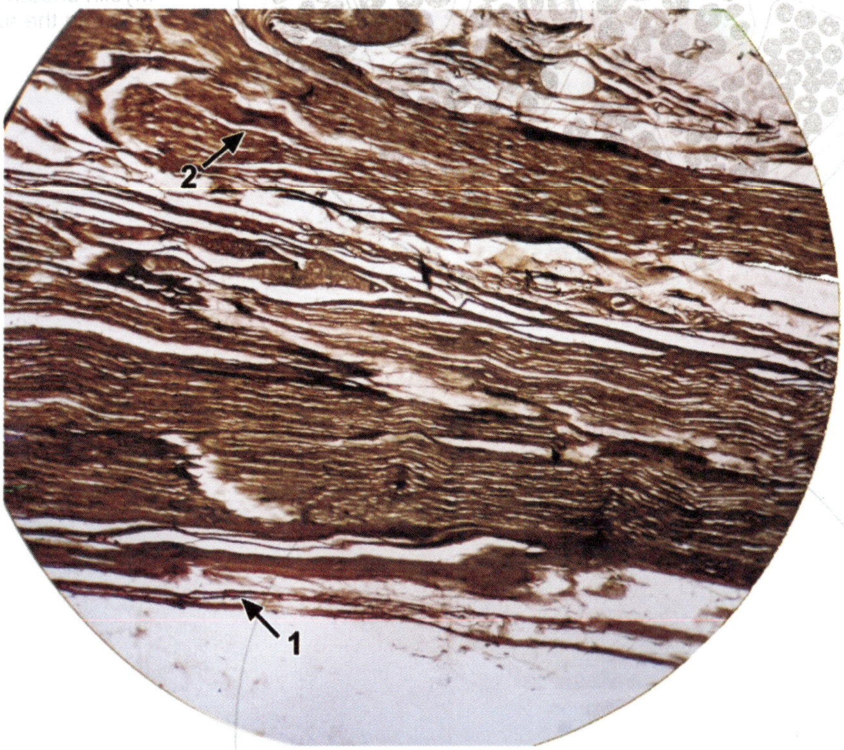

1. Perineurium
2. Myelin sheath around the axon

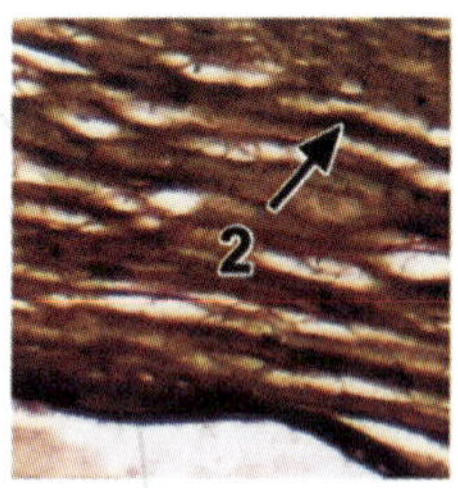

Key Features to Identify the Slide

[Osmic acid stain]

- Long and vertically arranged nerve fibres
- Centrally placed axon
- Myelin sheath with nodes of Ranvier

Examples

- Radial nerve
- Sciatic nerve

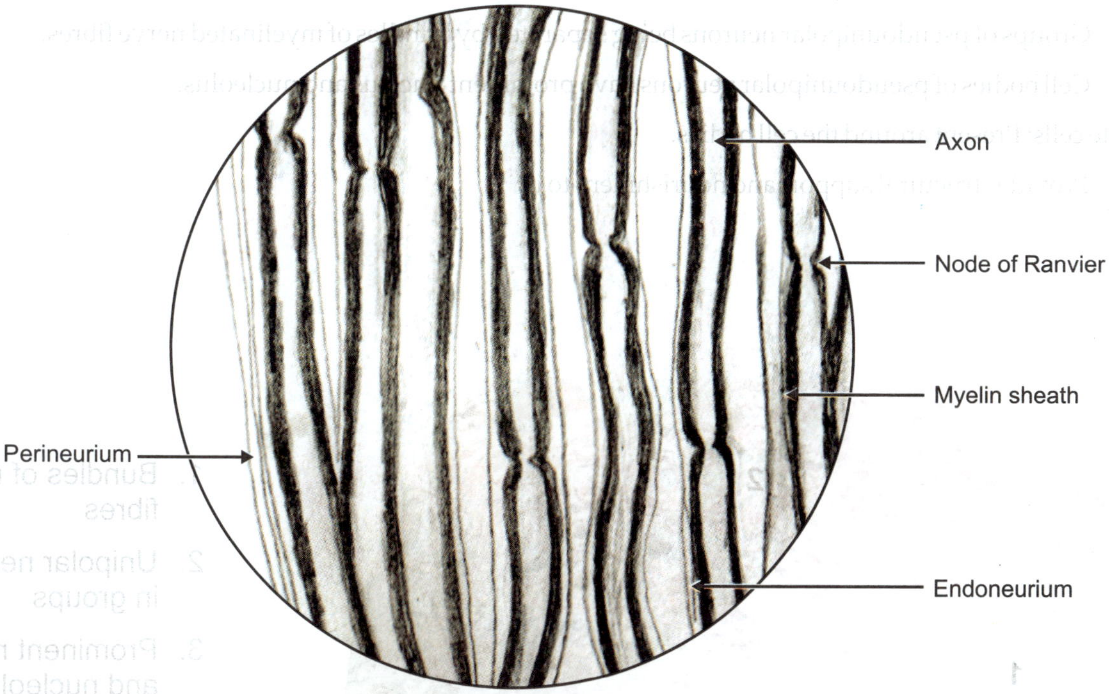
Axon
Node of Ranvier
Myelin sheath
Perineurium
Endoneurium

SENSORY (SPINAL) GANGLION

Ganglion: Collection of nerve cell bodies outside the central nervous system.

- Ganglion is covered by connective tissue capsule.
- Groups of pseudounipolar neurons being separated by bundles of myelinated nerve fibres.
- Cell bodies of pseudounipolar neurons have prominent nucleus and nucleolus.

Satellite cells: Present around the cell bodies.

- Provide structural support and nourishment to it.

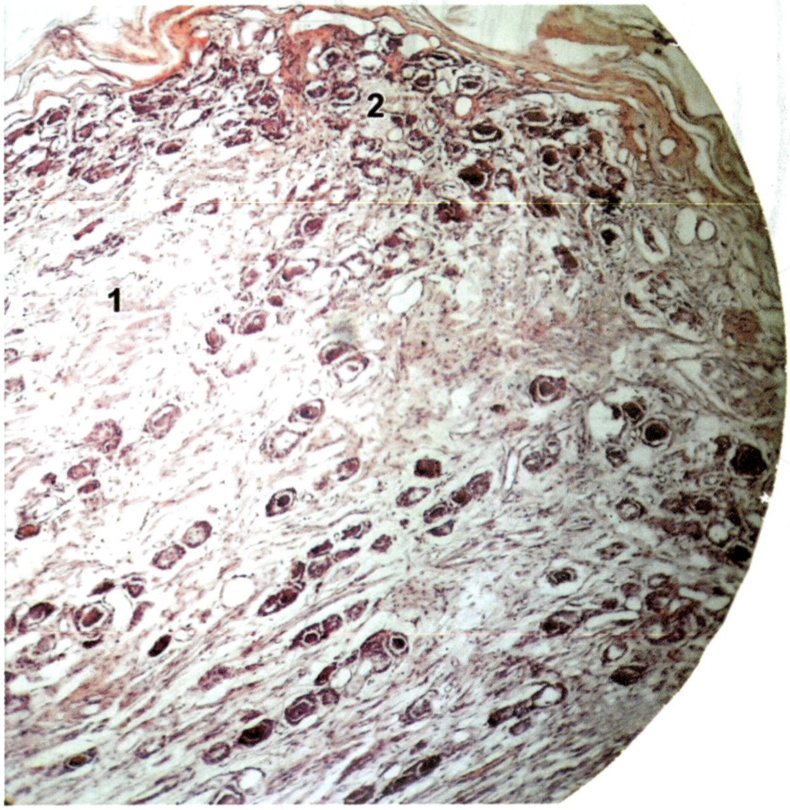

1. Bundles of nerve fibres
2. Unipolar neurons in groups
3. Prominent nucleus and nucleolus
4. Satellite cell

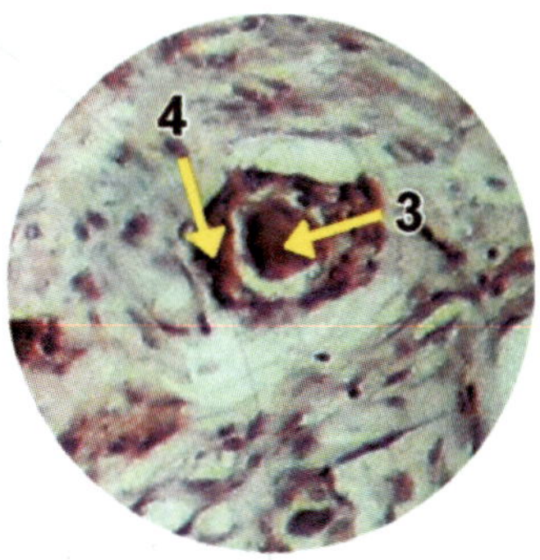

Key Features to Identify the Slide

- Presence of pseudounipolar neurons arranged in groups
- Centrally-placed nucleus
- Well-arranged satellite cells

Example

- Dorsal root ganglion/ spinal ganglion

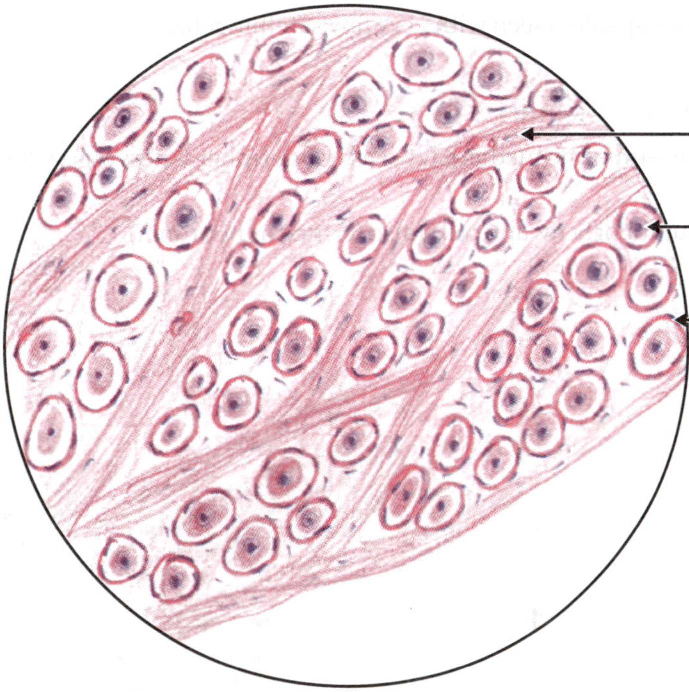
Nerve fibres
Ganglion cells
(pseudounipolar)
Satellite cells

AUTONOMIC (SYMPATHETIC) GANGLION

- Presence of numerous blood vessels in between the scattered cell bodies of multipolar neurons.
- Bundles of myelinated and non-myelinated nerve fibres run in between the nerve cell bodies.
- Thin connective tissue capsule is seen with very few satellite cells.

Applied Aspects of Nervous Tissue

1. Guillain-Barre syndrome—immune mediated disease of peripheral nervous system leading to demyelination of nerve fibres.
2. Schwannoma—benign tumor of Schwann cells (also termed as neuroma).

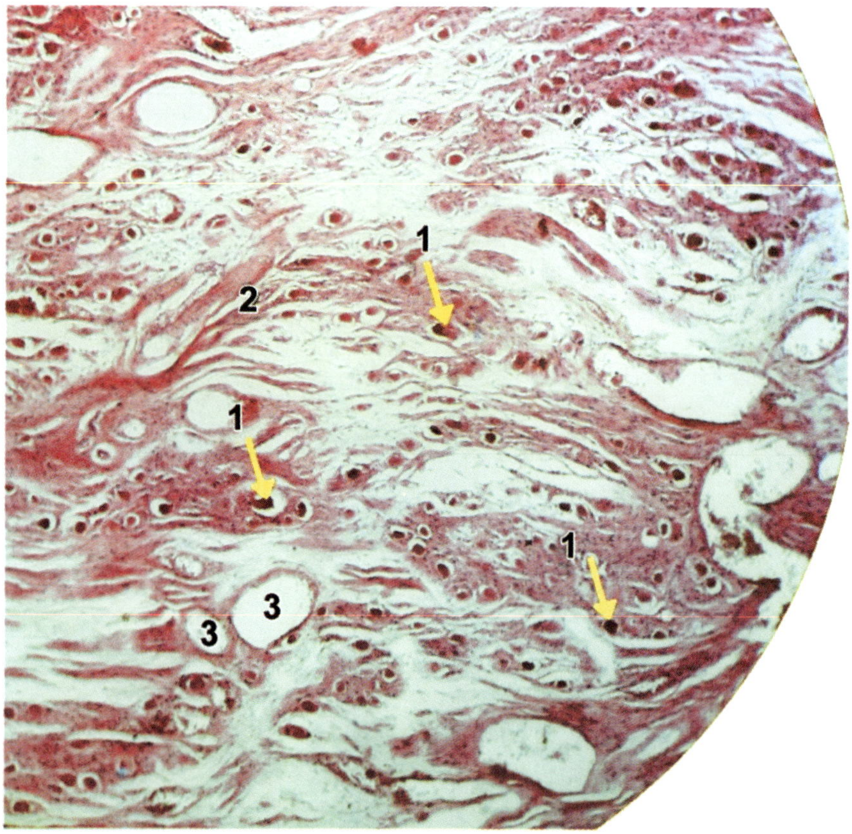

1. Multipolar neurons scattered
2. Bundles of nerve fibres
3. Blood vessels

Key Features to Identify the Slide

- Presence of scattered multipolar neurons
- Eccentrically placed nucleus
- Satellite cells are poorly defined

Example

– Superior cervical sympathetic ganglion

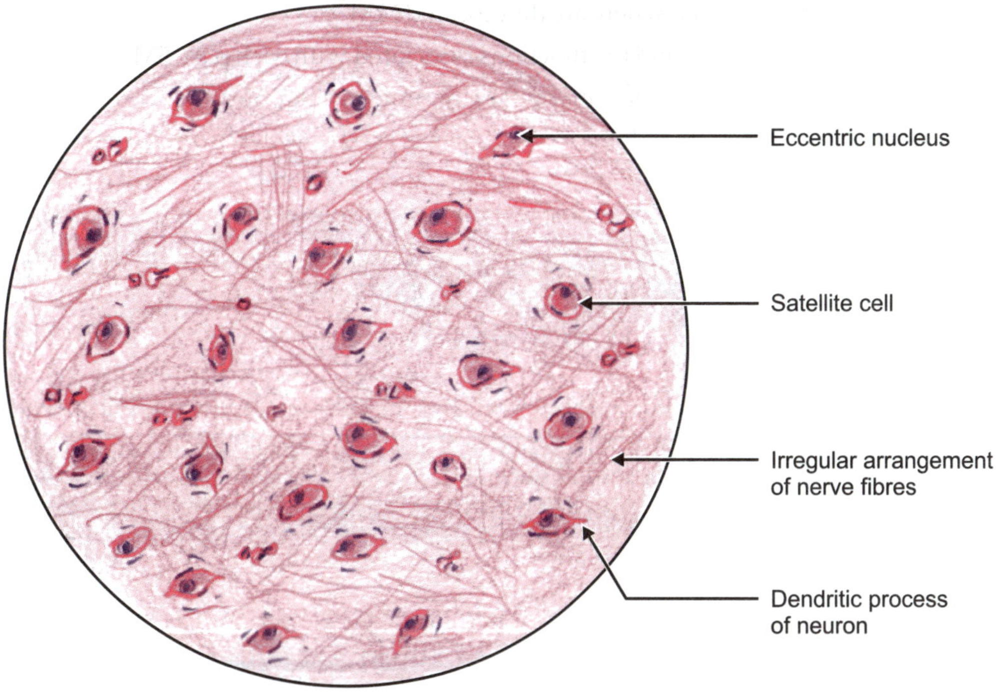
Eccentric nucleus
Satellite cell
Irregular arrangement of nerve fibres
Dendritic process of neuron

QUESTIONS

1. Explain neurilemma and its role in nerve function. 5M
2. Provide an overview of the structure of a neuron, including its main components and their functions. 5M
3. What are Nissl bodies and where are they located? 2M
4. Components of a neuron and the functions associated with each part. 5M
5. Microscopic characteristics of spinal and autonomic ganglia. 5M
6. Highlight the distinctions in the myelination process between the central nervous system (CNS) and peripheral nervous system (PNS). 5M
7. Enumerate the different types of neurons and give examples for each classification.5M
8. Name the various types of glial cells and elaborate on their respective functions. 5M
9. Elucidate the function of satellite cells in the nervous system. 2M

Figures/Notes

LARGE-SIZED ARTERY (ELASTIC ARTERY)

Functionally they are conducting vessels with the presence of following layers:

Tunica intima: Made up of endothelium (simple squamous epithelium), subendothelial connective tissue with few smooth muscle cells and internal elastic lamina.

- In large arteries internal elastic lamina cannot be differentiated as it merges with the elastic fibres of tunica media.

Tunica media: Made up of many layers of fenestrated sheaths of elastic fibres. It also contains few smooth muscle cells in between the elastic fibres.

- Presence of external elastic lamina outside the layer of elastic fibres (not prominent)

Tunica adventitia: Made up of connective tissue, rich in collagen fibres. There is also presence of few elastic fibres and connective tissue cells.

Vasa vasorum: Blood vessels supplying blood vessels are noticed which provide nutrition to the vessel wall.

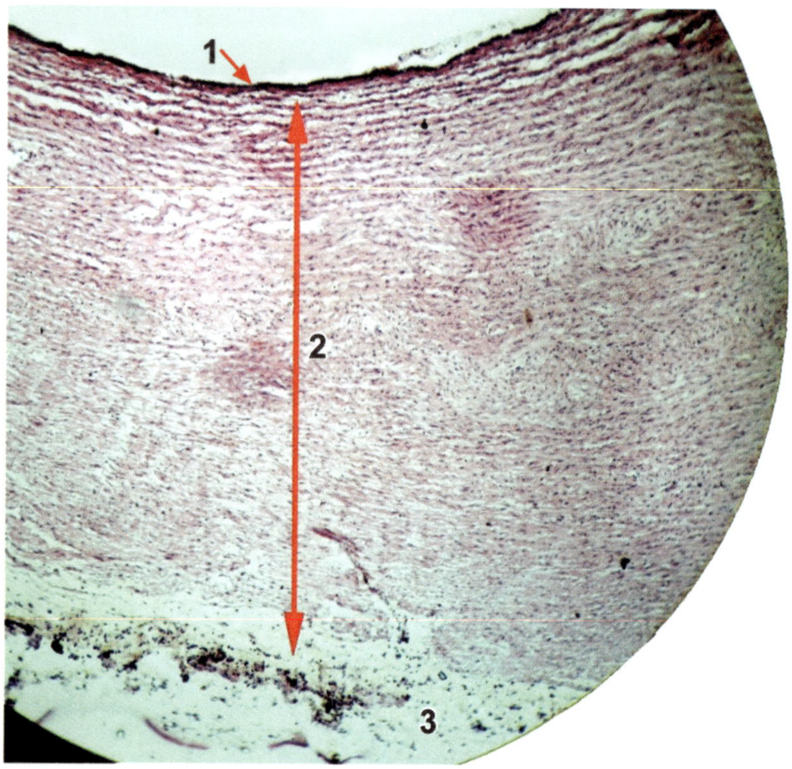

1. Tunica intima with endothelium, subendothelial connective tissue and internal elastic lamina
2. Tunica media
3. Tunica adventitia

Key Features to Identify the Slide

- Innermost tunica intima with endothelium and subendothelial connective tissue
- Tunica media is thick
- More number of elastic fibres in tunica media
- Vasa vasorum in tunica adventitia

Examples

- Aorta
- Brachiocephalic trunk

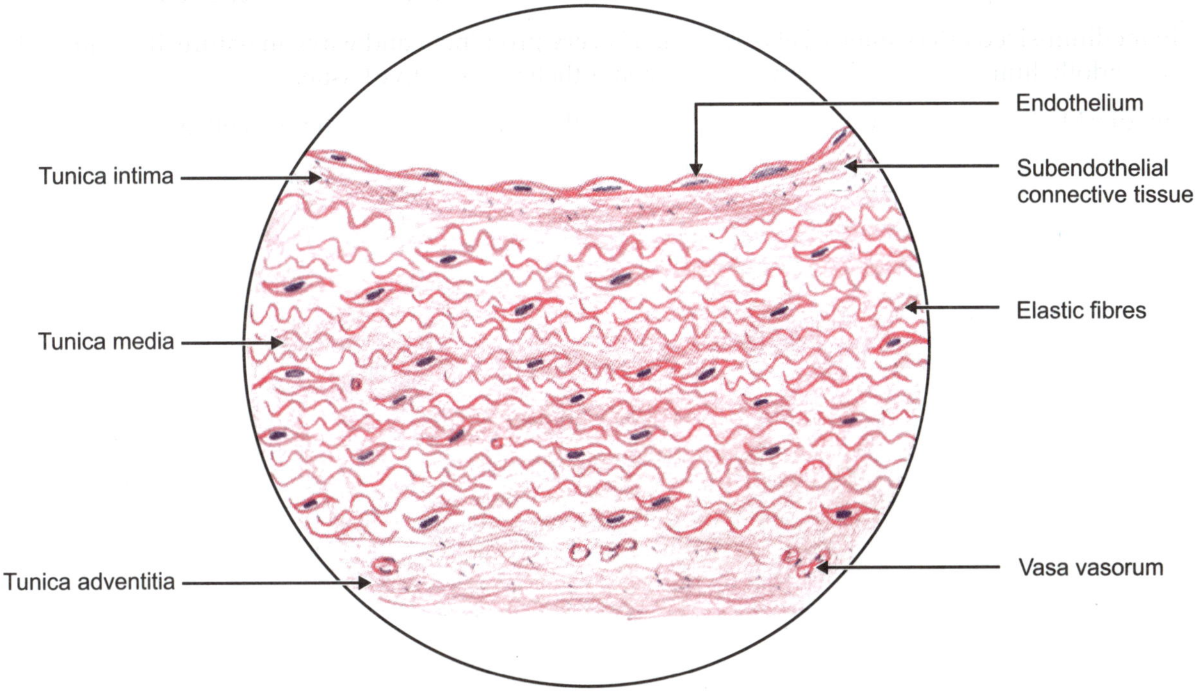
Endothelium
Tunica intima
Subendothelial connective tissue
Elastic fibres
Tunica media
Vasa vasorum
Tunica adventitia

MEDIUM-SIZED ARTERY (MUSCULAR ARTERY)

Functionally they are distributing arteries with the presence of following layers:

Tunica intima: Made up of endothelium, subendothelial connective tissue and internal elastic lamina.

- In medium-sized artery internal elastic lamina is very prominent and wavy in nature. It lies just adjacent to the endothelium because of less amount of subendothelial connective tissue.

Tunica media: Made up of layers of smooth muscle cells with less number of elastic and collagen fibres.

- Thin layer of external elastic lamina is visible in the region between the tunica media and tunica adventitia.

Tunica adventitia: Made up of connective tissue. It is thicker than tunica adventitia of large artery.

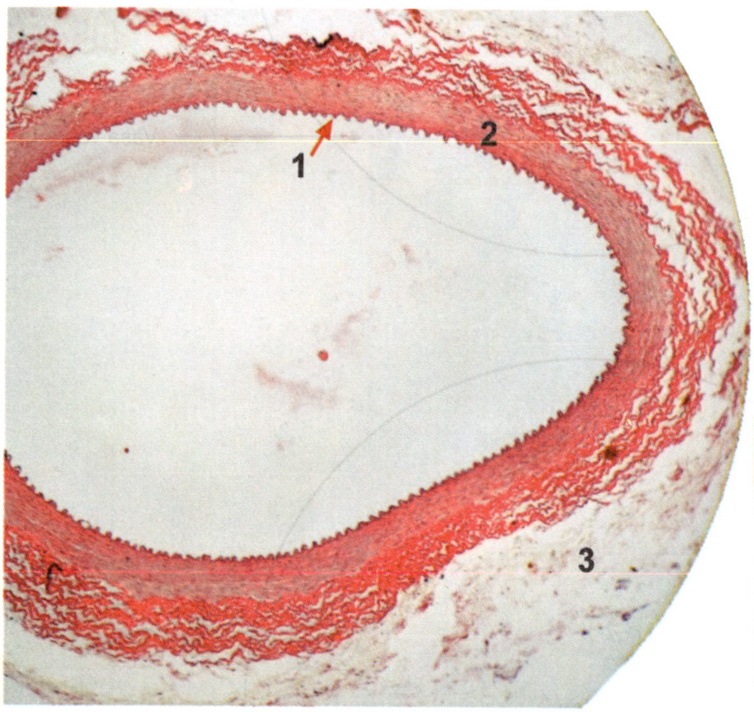

1. Wavy internal elastic lamina
2. Tunica media
3. Tunica adventitia

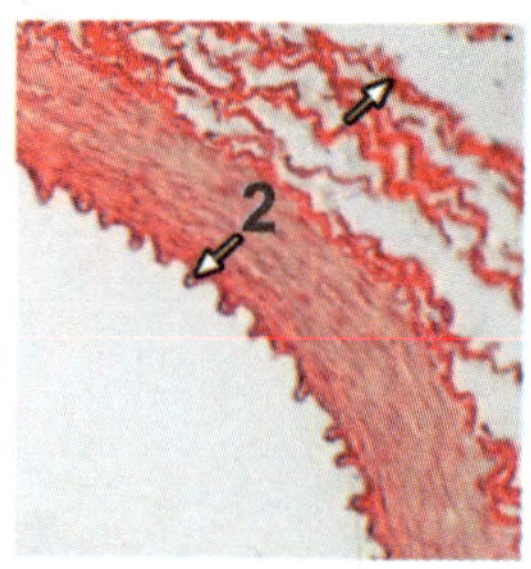

Key Features to Identify the Slide

- Prominent internal elastic lamina
- Thickest tunica media with more number of smooth muscle fibres in it
- Tunica adventitia predominantly made up of collagen fibres

Examples

- Radial artery
- Ulnar artery

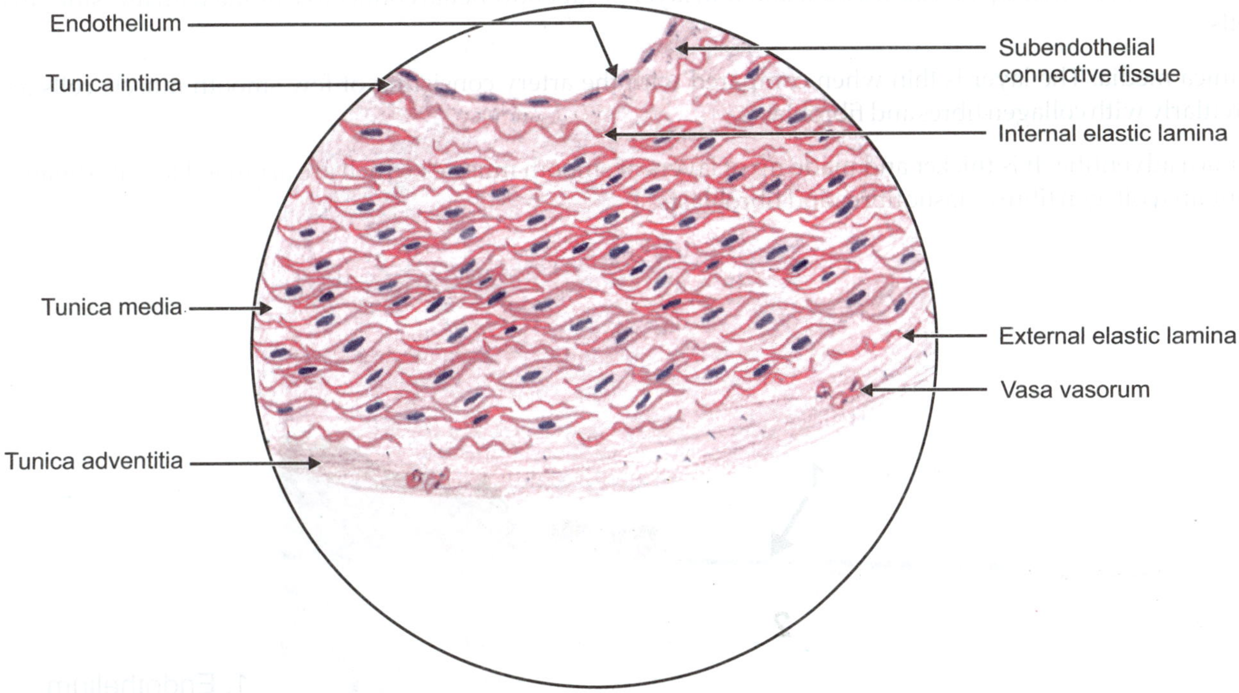
Endothelium
Tunica intima
Subendothelial connective tissue
Internal elastic lamina
Tunica media
External elastic lamina
Vasa vasorum
Tunica adventitia

LARGE-SIZED VEIN

Functionally they are reservoir vessels with the presence of following layers:

Tunica intima: Made up of endothelium and thin layer of subendothelial connective tissue with few smooth muscle cells.

Tunica media: The layer is thin when compared with the artery consisting of few smooth muscle cells arranged circularly with collagen fibres and fibroblasts.

Tunica adventitia: It is thicker and made up of layers of smooth muscles which are arranged longitudinally. It also contains collagen fibres, elastic fibres and fibroblasts.

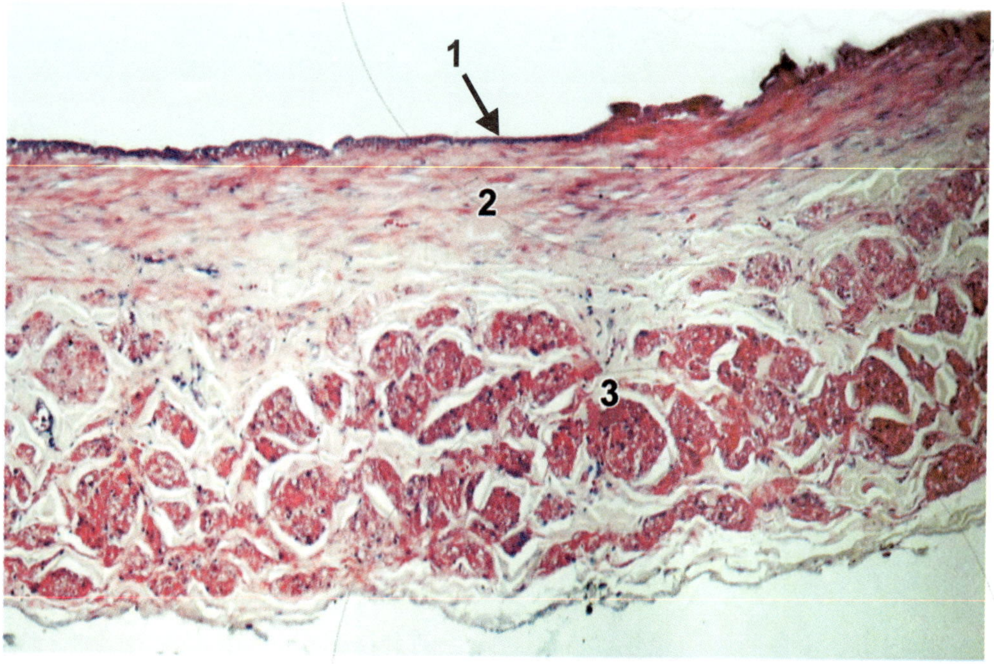

1. Endothelium
2. Tunica media
3. Muscle fibres (TS) of tunica adventitia

Key Features to Identify the Slide

- Lumen is collapsed
- Internal elastic lamina ill-defined
- Thick tunica adventitia with longitudinal bundles of smooth muscle fibres

Examples

- Superior vena cava
- Inferior vena cava

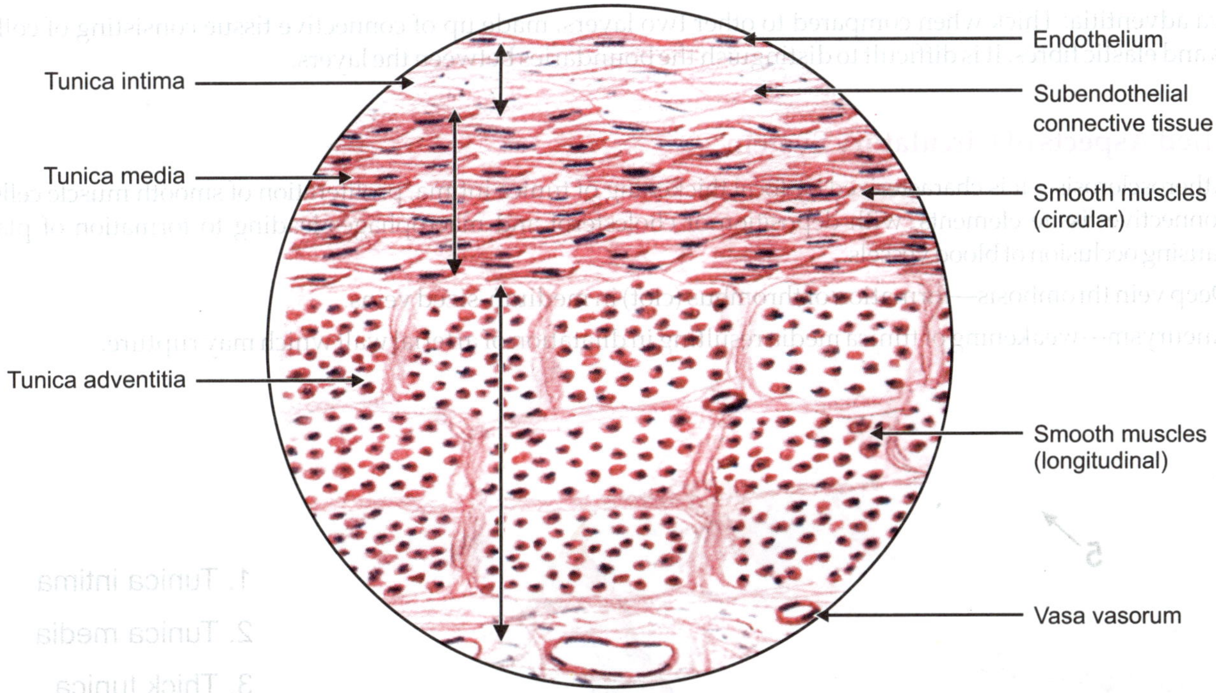
Endothelium
Tunica intima
Subendothelial connective tissue
Tunica media
Smooth muscles (circular)
Tunica adventitia
Smooth muscles (longitudinal)
Vasa vasorum

MEDIUM-SIZED VEIN

Tunica intima: It is very thin and made up of endothelium and subendothelial connective tissue.

Tunica media: It is thin, consists of few layers of smooth muscle cells.

Tunica adventitia: Thick when compared to other two layers, made up of connective tissue consisting of collagen fibres and elastic fibres. It is difficult to distinguish the boundaries between the layers.

Applied Aspects of Circulatory System

1. Atherosclerosis—it is characterized by focal thickening of tunica intima, proliferation of smooth muscle cells and connective tissue elements, with deposition of cholesterol and macrophages leading to formation of plaques causing occlusion of blood vessels.
2. Deep vein thrombosis—formation of thrombus (clot) in medium-sized veins.
3. Aneurysm—weakening of tunica media resulting in dilatation of arterial wall which may rupture.

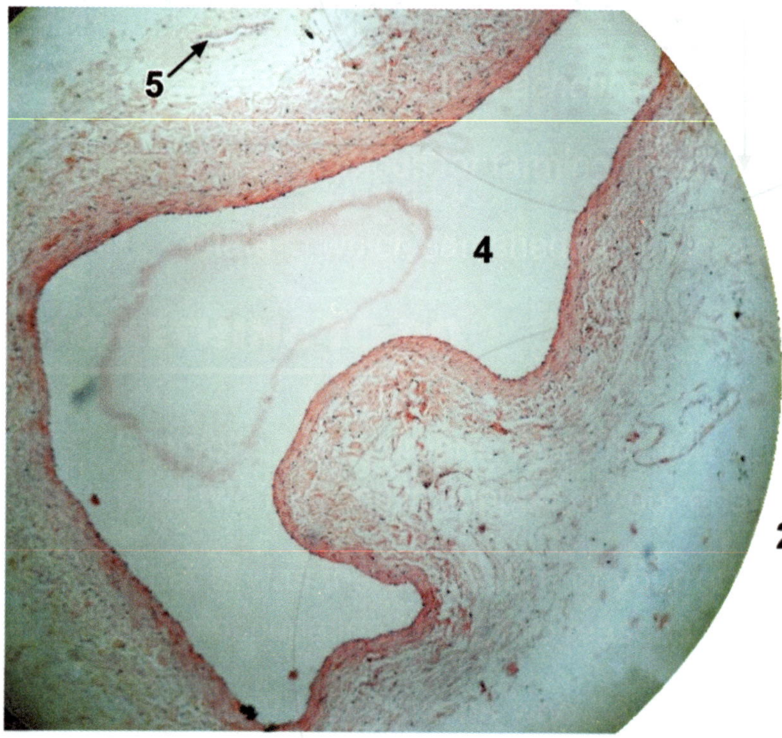

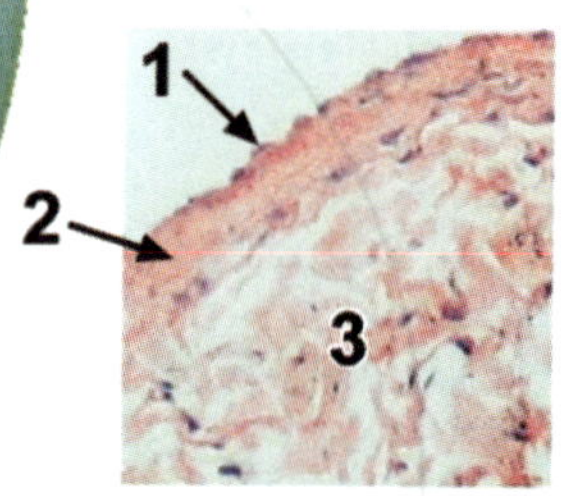

1. Tunica intima
2. Tunica media
3. Thick tunica adventitia
4. Collapsed lumen
5. Vasa vasorum

Key Features to Identify the Slide

- Large collapsed lumen
- Thin tunica media with a few circular smooth muscle fibres
- Thick tunica adventitia with dense irregular connective tissue fibres

Examples

- Cephalic vein
- Short saphenous vein

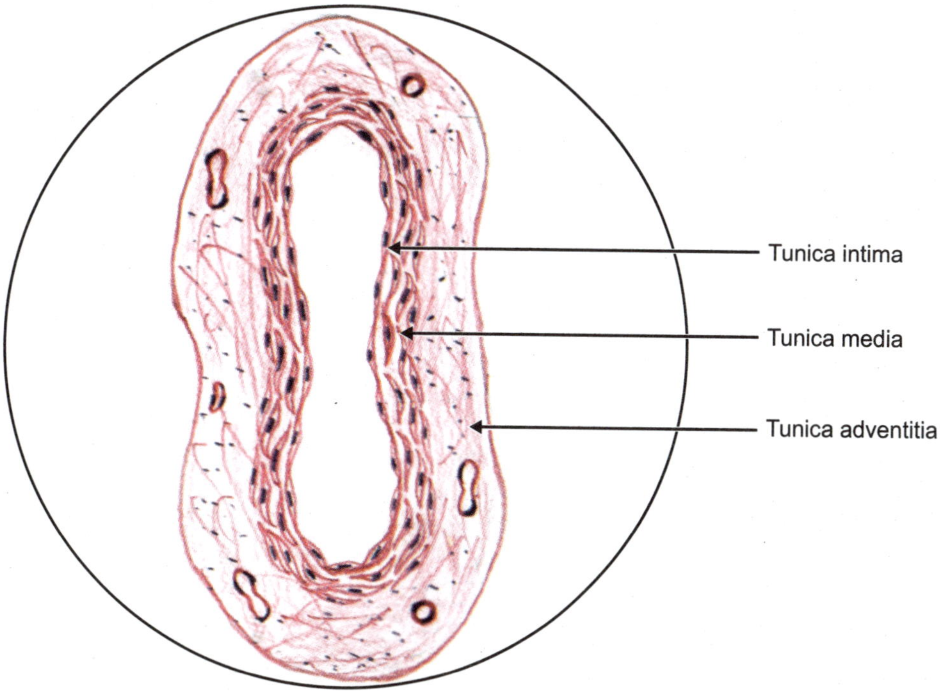
Tunica intima
Tunica media
Tunica adventitia

QUESTIONS

1. Define internal elastic lamina? 2M
2. Explain the histological difference between a large-sized artery and medium-sized artery? 5M
3. What is endothelium and its function? 2M
4. Brief about the general structure of a blood vessel. 2M
5. Name the different types of capillaries with examples. 2M
6. Compare the microscopic features of a large-sized artery and a large-sized vein. 5M
7. Compare the microscopic features of a medium-sized artery and a medium-sized vein. 5M

Figures/Notes

LYMPH NODE

Capsule: Made up of connective tissue, trabeculae extend from the capsule and enters the substance of the node which is supported by the meshwork of reticular tissue.

- Presence of subcapsular sinus beneath the capsule.

Cortex: Consists of lymphatic nodules, some of them (secondary lymphatic nodules) exhibiting outer dark zone of densely packed lymphocytes and inner lightly stained germinal centre filled with large lymphoblasts.

- Lymphatic nodule contains mainly B-lymphocytes and paracortex contains T- lymphocytes.

Medulla: Presence of anastomosing cords of cells like lymphocytes, macrophages, plasma cells and few antigen presenting cells.

- In between the medullary cords there are sinuses through which the circulation of lymph occurs.

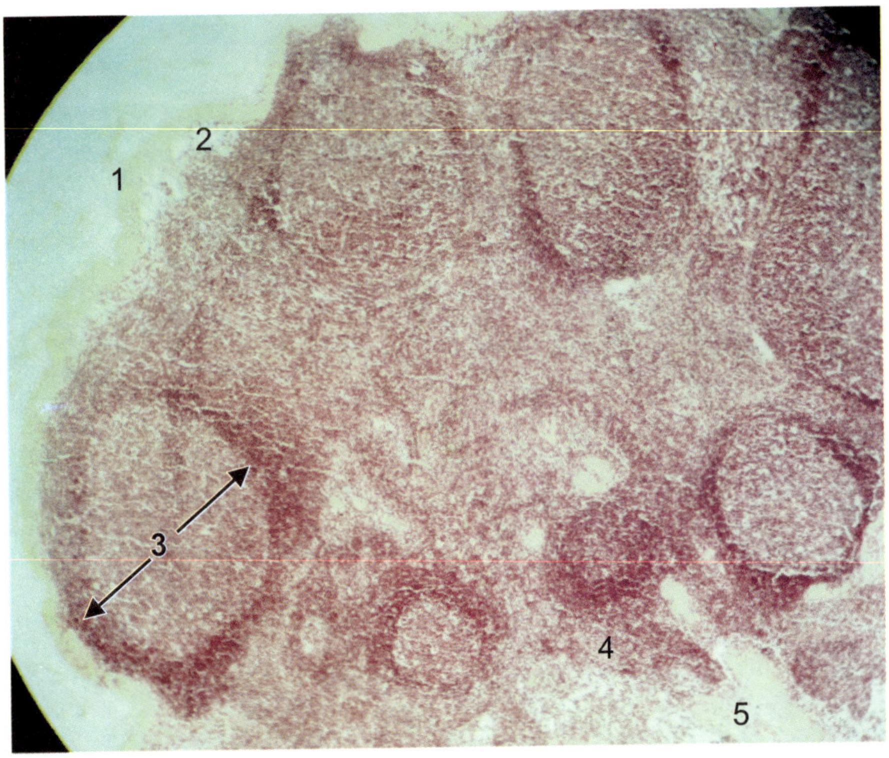

1. Capsule
2. Subcapsular sinus
3. Cortial lymphatic nodule with germinal centre
4. Medullary cords
5. Medullary sinus

Key Features to Identify the Slide

- Thin capsule around the node
- Presence of lymphatic nodules in cortex
- Presence of subcapsular sinus
- Medullary cords and sinuses present in medulla

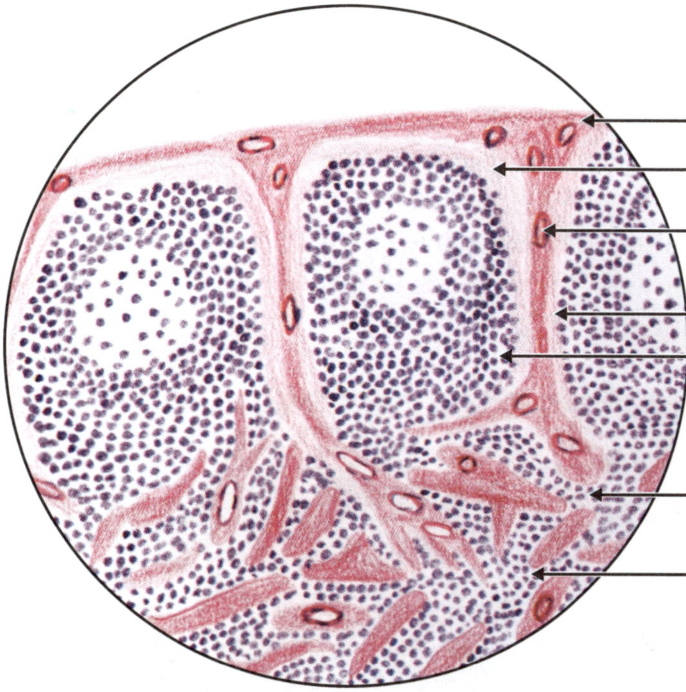
Capsule
Subcapsular sinus
Trabeculum with capillary
Trabecular sinus
Cortical nodule
Medullary cords
Medullary sinus

SPLEEN

Capsule: Consists of dense connective tissue.

- Incomplete trabeculae arise from the capsule and enter into the parenchyma of spleen.

White pulp: Consists of lymphatic follicles with germinal centre in some of the follicles. These follicles are called Malpighian corpuscles. They have eccentric arteriole.

- As it is the central artery which is pushed to the periphery it is termed as periarteriolar lymphatic sheath (PALS).

Red pulp: Made up of anastomosing network of splenic cords of cells (cords of billroth) containing B-lymphocytes, T- lymphocytes, macrophages, plasma cells and erythrocytes.

- In between them are sinusoids lined by endothelial cells called stave cells.

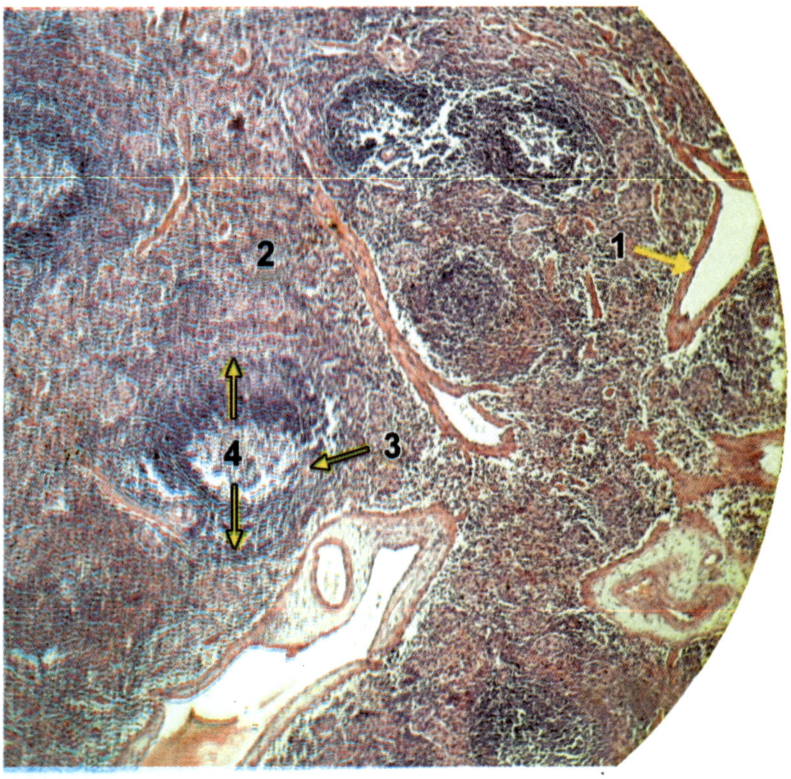

1. Trabeculae
2. Red pulp
3. Central arteriole
4. Lymphatic nodule (white pulp)

Key Features to Identify the Slide

- Thick capsule with trabeculae
- Presence of red pulp and white pulp
- Eccentrically placed artery in white pulp
- Red pulp with splenic cords and sinusoids

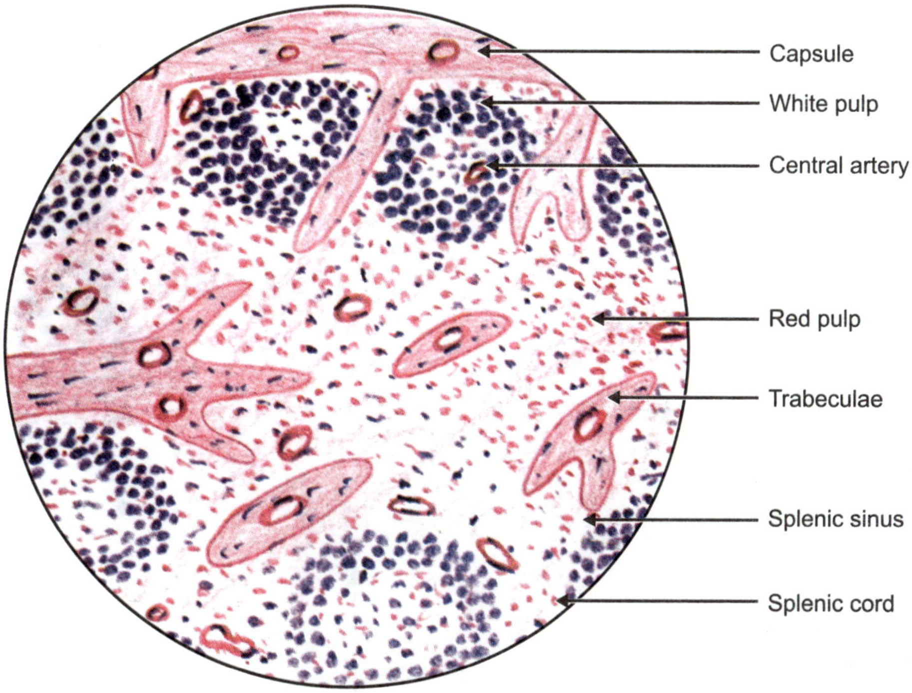
Capsule
White pulp
Central artery
Red pulp
Trabeculae
Splenic sinus
Splenic cord

THYMUS

Capsule: Made up of connective tissue, septa arise from the capsule and divide the gland into incomplete lobules.

- Lymphocytes in the thymus are supported by meshwork of epithelio-reticular cells (epitheliocytes)
- Lobules made up of outer cortex and inner medulla.

Cortex: Darkly stained due to closely packed T-lymphocytes.

Medulla: It is lightly stained due to less dense arrangement of lymphoblasts and lymphocytes.

- Medulla contains circumscribed eosinophilic structures called Hassall's corpuscles. They are concentrically arranged epitheliocytes around degenerated mass.

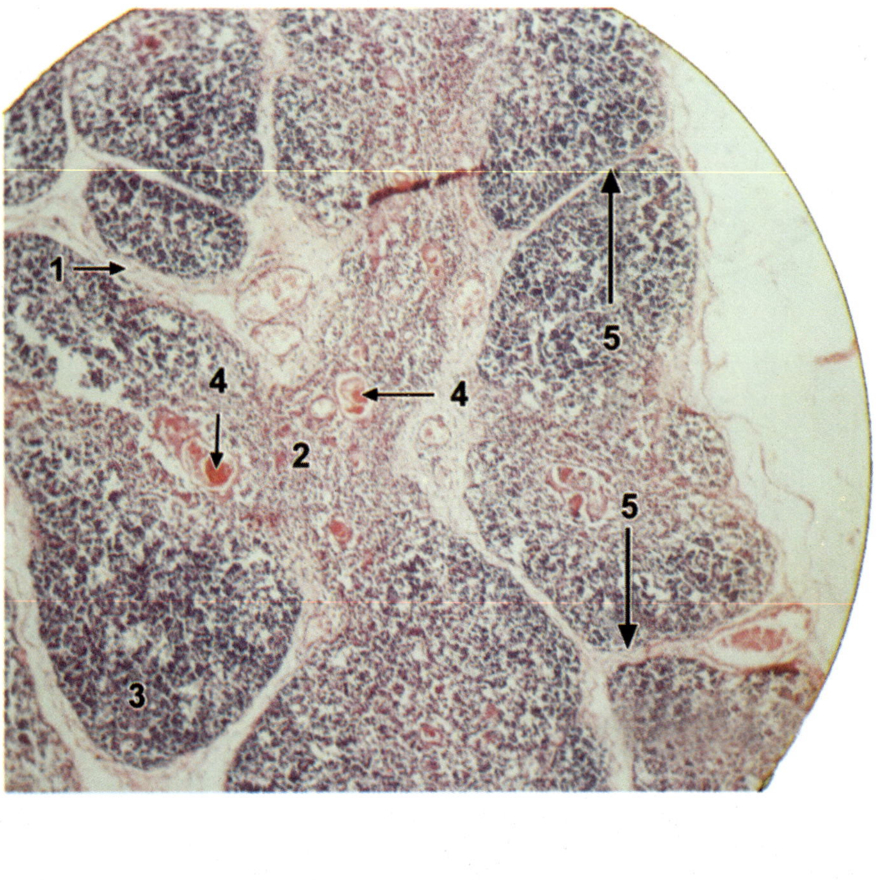

1. Trabeculae
2. Medulla
3. Cortex
4. Thymic (Hassall's corpuscles)
5. Lobule

Key Features to Identify the Slide

- Presence of lobules with incomplete septae
- Cortex and medulla in each lobule
- Presence of Hassall's corpuscles in medulla

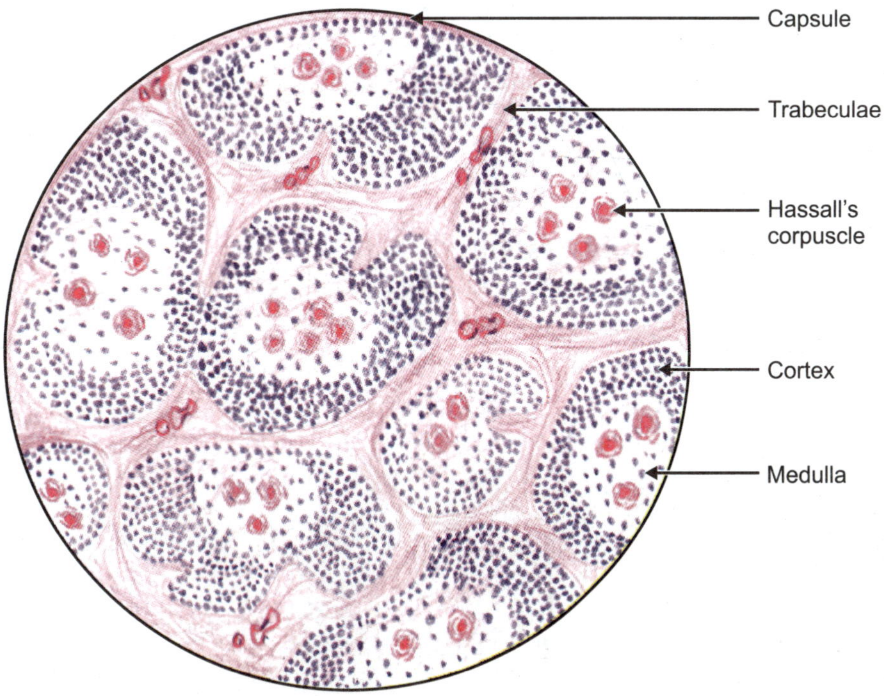
Capsule
Trabeculae
Hassall's corpuscle
Cortex
Medulla

PALATINE TONSIL

Tonsillar crypts: Stratified squamous non-keratinized epithelium lining the surface of the tonsil, invaginate into the substance as crypts.

Lymphatic nodules: As lymphatic nodules are present beneath the mucosa it is classified as mucosa associated lymphoid tissue (MALT).

- Some nodules possess germinal centre indicating the exposure of antigen to it.
- Nodules contain both B and T lymphocytes being supported by meshwork of reticular tissue.
- Collection of mucus acini are noticed beneath the epithelium.

Applied Aspects of Lymphoid System

1. Reactive (inflammatory) lymphadenitis—enlargement of lymph nodes because of hyperplasia of lymphatic nodules secondary to bacterial and other microbial infections.
2. Thymoma— enlargement of thymus gland which can be benign or malignant.

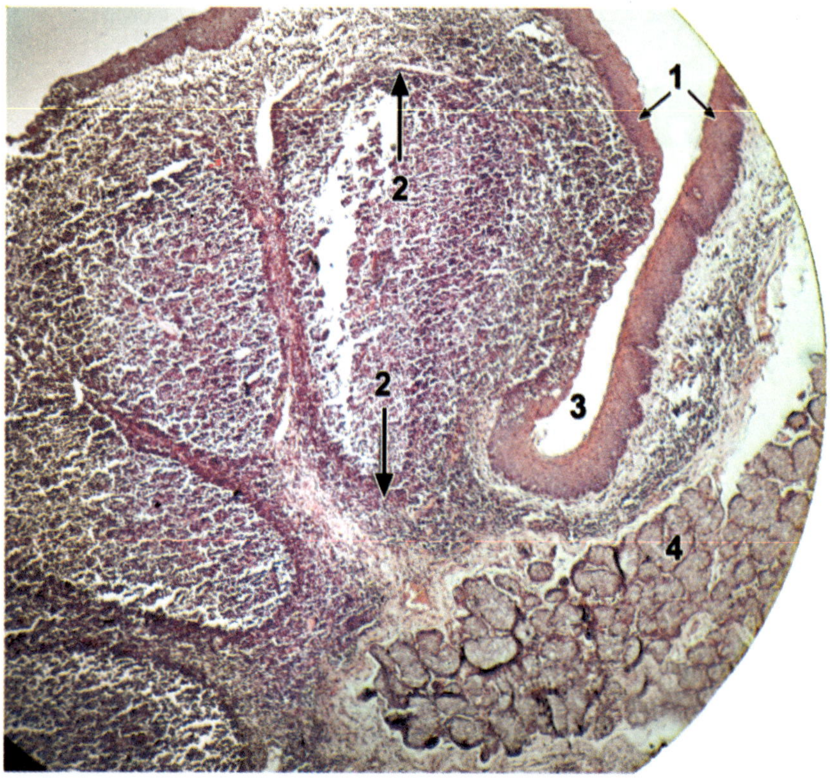

1. Stratified squamous non-keratinized epithelium
2. Lymphatic nodule
3. Tonsillar crypt
4. Mucous glands

Key Features to Identify the Slide

- Deep tonsillar crypt is seen
- Stratified squamous non-keratinized epithelium
- Presence of lymphatic nodules just below the epithelium

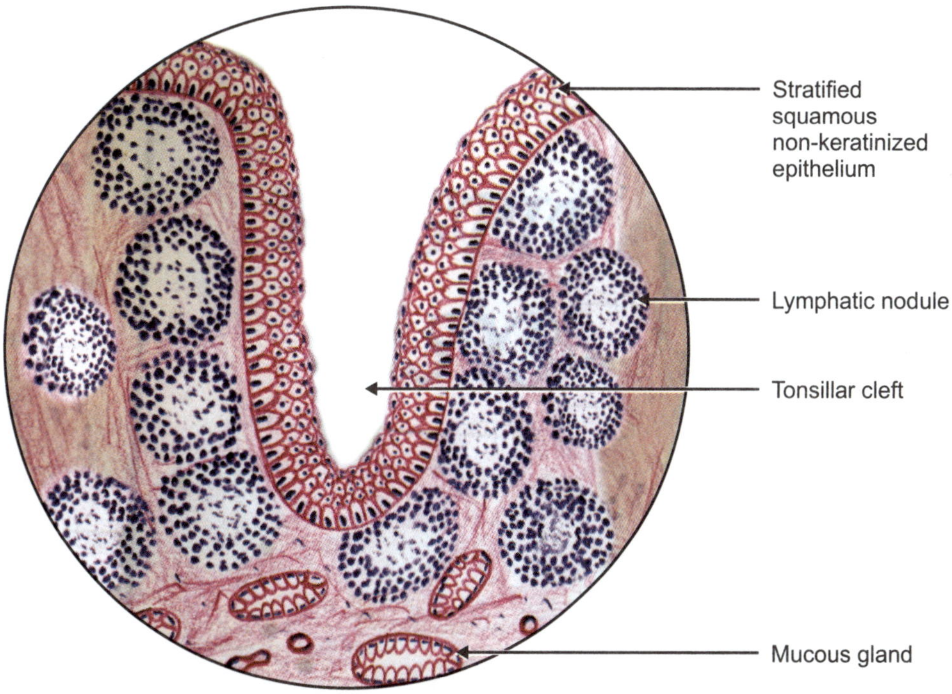
Stratified squamous non-keratinized epithelium
Lymphatic nodule
Tonsillar cleft
Mucous gland

QUESTIONS

1. Mention the functions of spleen. 2M
2. Provide an in-depth explanation of splenic circulation, emphasizing the constituents of red and white pulp within the spleen. 5M
3. Discuss the histology of lymph node. 5M
4. Classify lymphoid organs and provide a detailed account of the microscopic anatomy of the thymus. 5M
5. Define lymphatic nodule. 2M
6. Enumerate the components of the medulla of a lymph node? 2M
7. What are Hassall's corpuscles? 2M
8. What are the types of lymphocytes in the outer and deep cortex of lymph node? 2M
9. Write the functions of lymph node? 2M
10. Define germinal centre of the lymphatic nodule. 2M

Figures/Notes

EPIGLOTTIS

- Anterior and upper part of posterior surface is lined by stratified squamous non-keratinized epithelium
- Posterior surface is lined by pseudostratified ciliated columnar epithelium (respiratory epithelium)
- Lamina propria underneath both the epithelium is made up of connective tissue containing serous and mucous glands
- A central part of elastic cartilage with perichondrium provides skeletal framework to the epiglottis

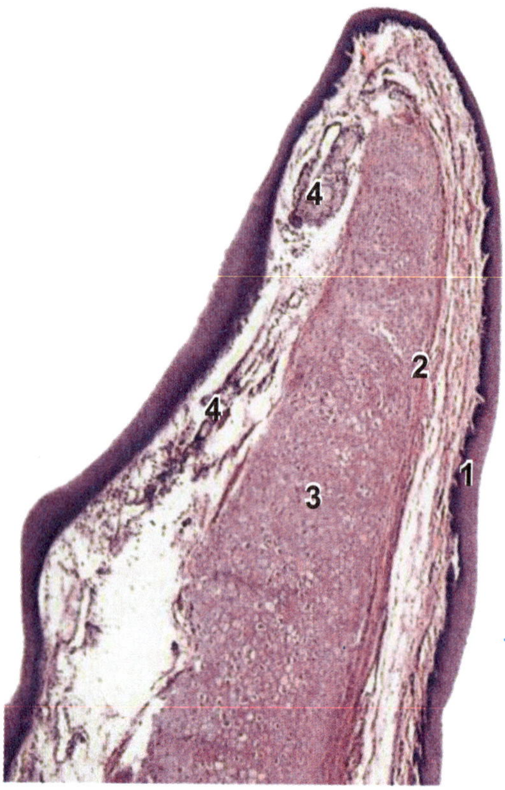

1. Stratified squamous non-keratinized epithelium
2. Perichondrium
3. Elastic cartilage
4. Seromucous glands

Key Features to Identify the Slide

- Anterior (lingual) surface is lined by stratified squamous non-keratinized epithelium
- Posterior (laryngeal) surface is lined by pseudostratified ciliated columnar epithelium with goblet cells
- In between is a plate of elastic cartilage

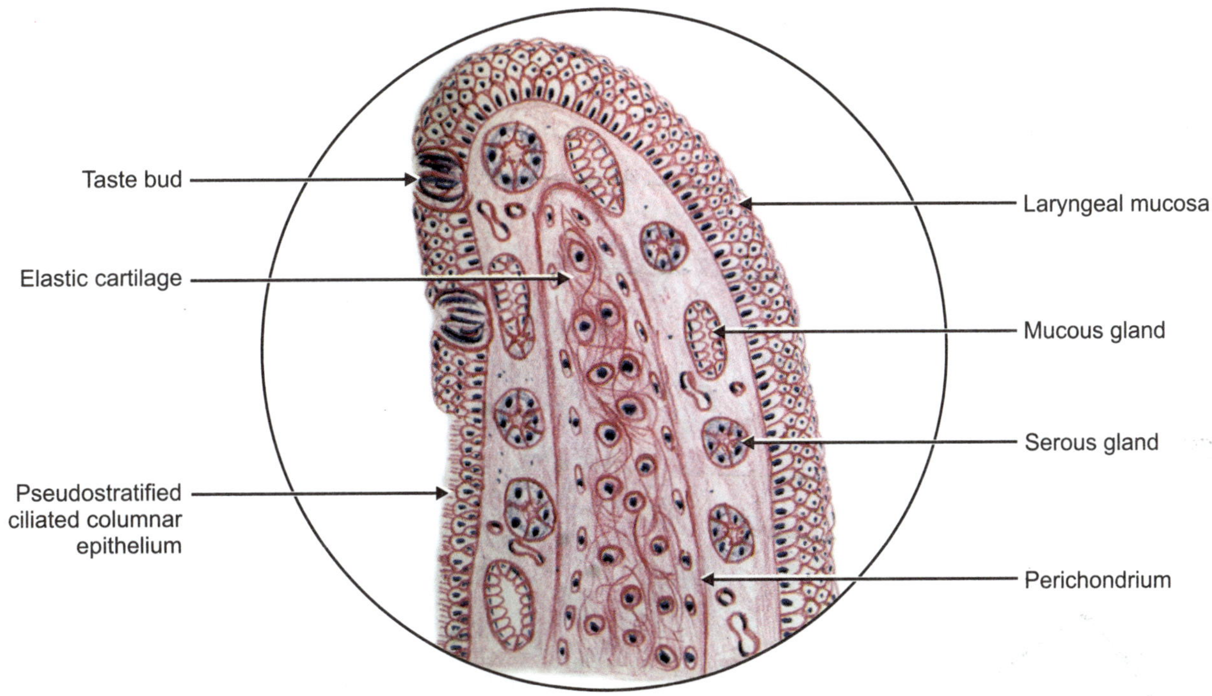
Taste bud
Elastic cartilage
Pseudostratified
ciliated columnar
epithelium
Laryngeal mucosa
Mucous gland
Serous gland
Perichondrium

TRACHEA

Wall of the trachea consists of following four layers:

1. Mucous membrane—lined by pseudostratified ciliated columnar epithelium with columnar cells, goblet cells, basal cells and small granule cells present in it.
   - Beneath the epithelium is lamina propria made up of loose connective tissue rich in elastic fibres.
   - Presence of BALT (bronchus associated lymphoid tissue) might be seen.
2. Submucosa—layers of connective tissue which contains mucus and serous glands along with blood vessels, nerves and lymphatics.
3. Cartilage and muscle layer—histological section of C-shaped hyaline cartilage is noticed beneath the submucosa.
   - It is covered by perichondrium and has typical features of hyaline cartilage.
   - The cartilage is incomplete posteriorly and the gap is filled by the presence of smooth muscles (trachealis muscle)

Adventitia: Layer of connective tissue made up of elastic fibres with blood vessels and nerves.

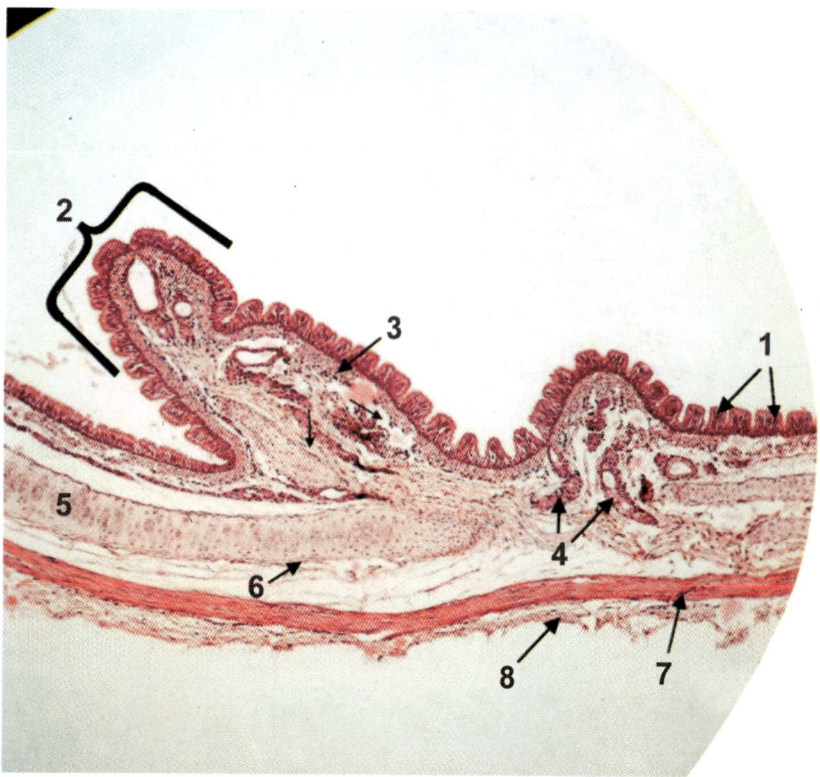

1. Pseudostratified ciliated columnar epithelium with goblet cell
2. Fold in tracheal mucosa
3. Lamina propria
4. Submucosa with glands
5. Tracheal cartilage (hyaline)
6. Perichondrium
7. Trachealis (smooth muscle)
8. Adventitia (fibrosa)

Key Features to Identify the Slide

- Pseudostratified ciliated columnar epithelium with goblet cells
- Serous and mucous glands in submucosa
- Presence of hyaline cartilage with perichondrium covering it

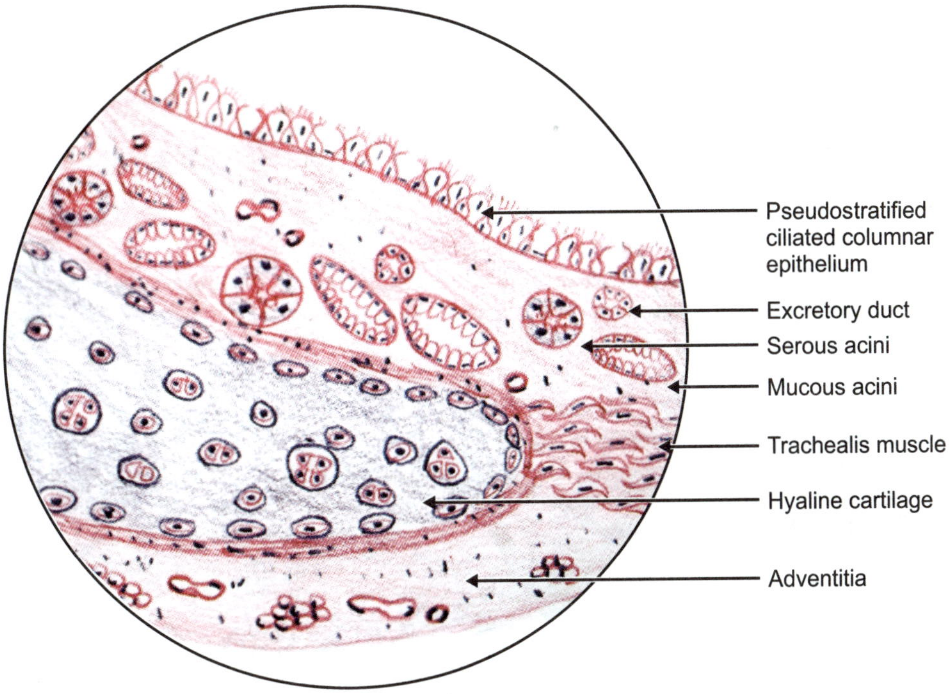
Pseudostratified ciliated columnar epithelium
Excretory duct
Serous acini
Mucous acini
Trachealis muscle
Hyaline cartilage
Adventitia

LUNG

Histological section of the lung includes—intrapulmonary bronchi, bronchioles and alveoli.

Intrapulmonary bronchus—made up of:

a. Mucosa—lined by pseudostratified ciliated columnar epithelium with goblet cells and layer of lamina propria beneath it.
b. Muscular layer—consists of bundles of smooth muscle fibres which are spirally arranged.
c. Submucosa—made up of loose connective tissue with seromucous glands.
d. Cartilage layer—presence of irregular plates of hyaline cartilage to keep the bronchi patent.
e. Adventitia—it is a layer of connective tissue containing blood vessels.

Bronchioles are conducting tubules less than 1 mm in diameter possessing following layers:

Mucosa: Lined by epithelium which varies from ciliated columnar epithelium to simple cuboidal epithelium depending upon its size.

- In smaller bronchioles goblet cells are replaced by Clara cells which secrete surfactant that reduce the surface tension of alveolar fluid and prevents the collapse of alveoli.

Smooth muscle layer: It is very prominent in bronchioles and innervated by autonomic nerve fibres. Connective tissue layer:

- This is thin layer of connective tissue made up of elastic fibres.

Note: Absence of hyaline cartilage and seromucous glands.

Alveoli: They are thin walled sacs lined by type I and type II pneumocytes.

Type I: Are simple squamous cells.

Type II: Are cuboidal cells which secrete surfactant.

- Alveoli are separated by interalveolar septa made up of small amount of connective tissue with capillaries. This is the basis of formation of blood air barrier.

Applied Aspects of Respiratory System

1. Bronchial asthma—chronic inflammatory disease involving airways characterized by recurrent obstruction of airflow because of inflammation of bronchioles and constriction of their smooth muscles (bronchospasm), due to combination of genetic and environmental factors.
2. Pneumonia—inflammation of alveoli of lung caused by various microorganisms

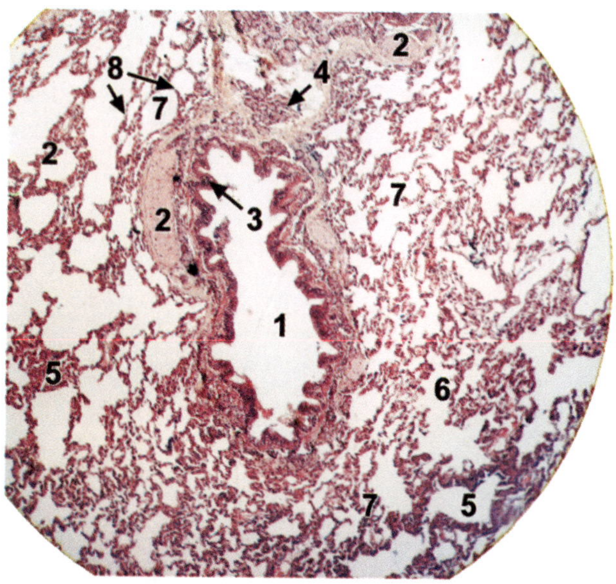

1. Lumen of intrapulmonary bronchus
2. Cartilage plate (hyaline)
3. Pseudostratified ciliated columnar epithelium
4. Seromucous gland
5. Respiratory bronchiole
6. Alveolar duct
7. Alveolar sac
8. Wall of alveoli (simple squamous epithelium)

Key Features to Identify the Slide

- Presence of alveoli giving honeycomb appearance
- Alveoli lined by simple squamous epithelium
- Intrapulmonary bronchi, terminal bronchioles and respiratory bronchioles are seen

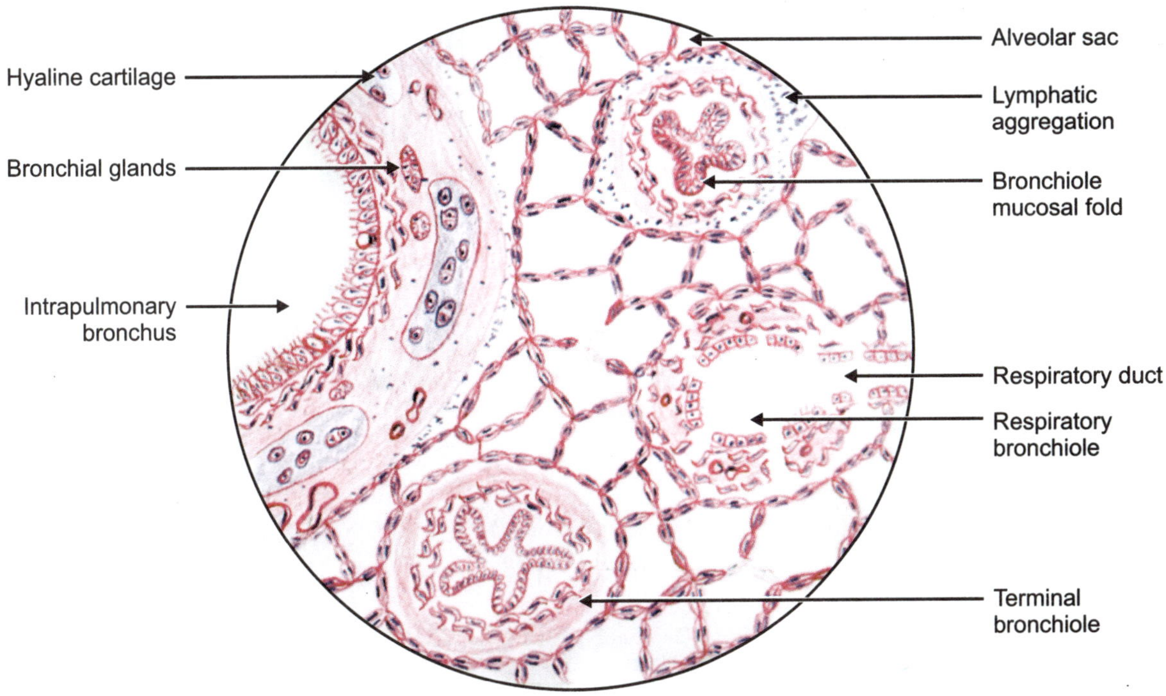
Hyaline cartilage
Bronchial glands
Intrapulmonary bronchus
Alveolar sac
Lymphatic aggregation
Bronchiole mucosal fold
Respiratory duct
Respiratory bronchiole
Terminal bronchiole

QUESTIONS

1. What are the types of cells present in the tracheal epithelium, and what are their respiratory functions? 2M
2. Define Clara cells and specify their location in the airway and their role in respiration. 2M
3. Highlight differences between respiratory bronchioles and terminal bronchioles. 2M
4. Write a short note on intrapulmonary bronchus. 5M
5. Define the conducting and respiratory parts of the respiratory tract and describe their collaborative functions. 5M
6. Summarize changes observed in epithelial and cartilaginous structures along the respiratory tract from trachea to alveoli and their impact on respiratory function. 5M
7. Microscopic structure of lung. 5M

Figures/Notes

11 Oral Cavity and Associated Structures (AN 43.2, 43.3, 70.1)

LIP

- External surface is lined by keratinized stratified squamous epithelium containing hair follicles, sweat glands and sebaceous glands.
- Internal surface lined by non-keratinized stratified squamous epithelium of the oral cavity. Connective tissue beneath the epithelium contains mucus secreting labial glands and blood vessels.
- The transition zone (red margin) of skin epidermis to oral epithelium is the region of mucocutaneous junction.
- The core of the lip contains striated muscle, orbicularis oris.

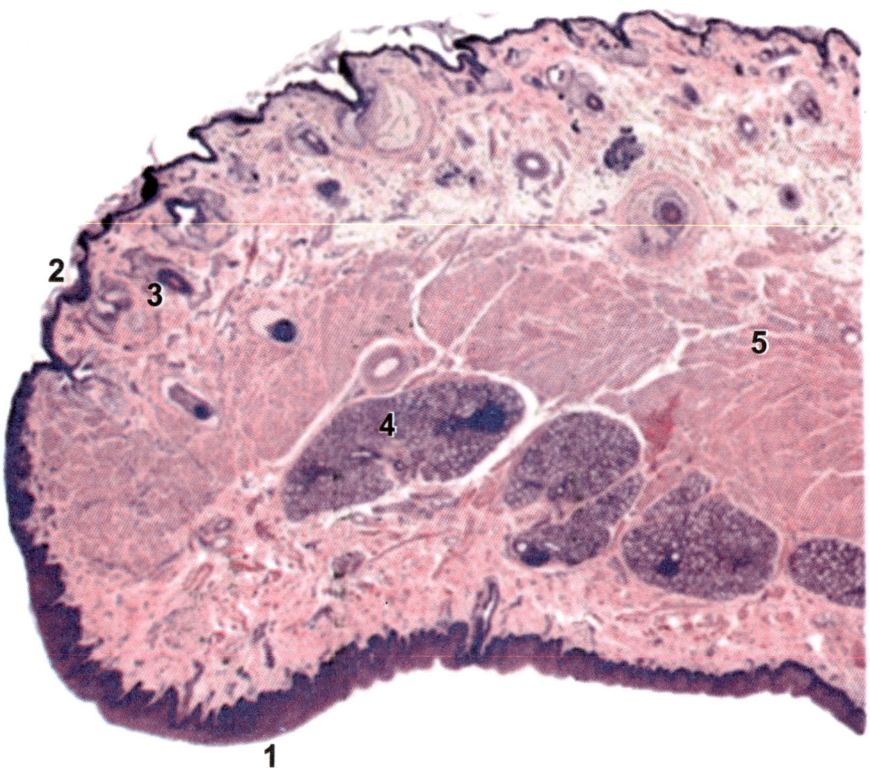

1. Oral epithelium
2. Transitional zone
3. Hair follicle
4. Mucous secretory glands
5. Orbicularis oris

Key Features to Identify the Slide

- External surface is covered by skin
- Internal surface is covered by mucous membrane
- Substance of the lip made up of skeletal muscle

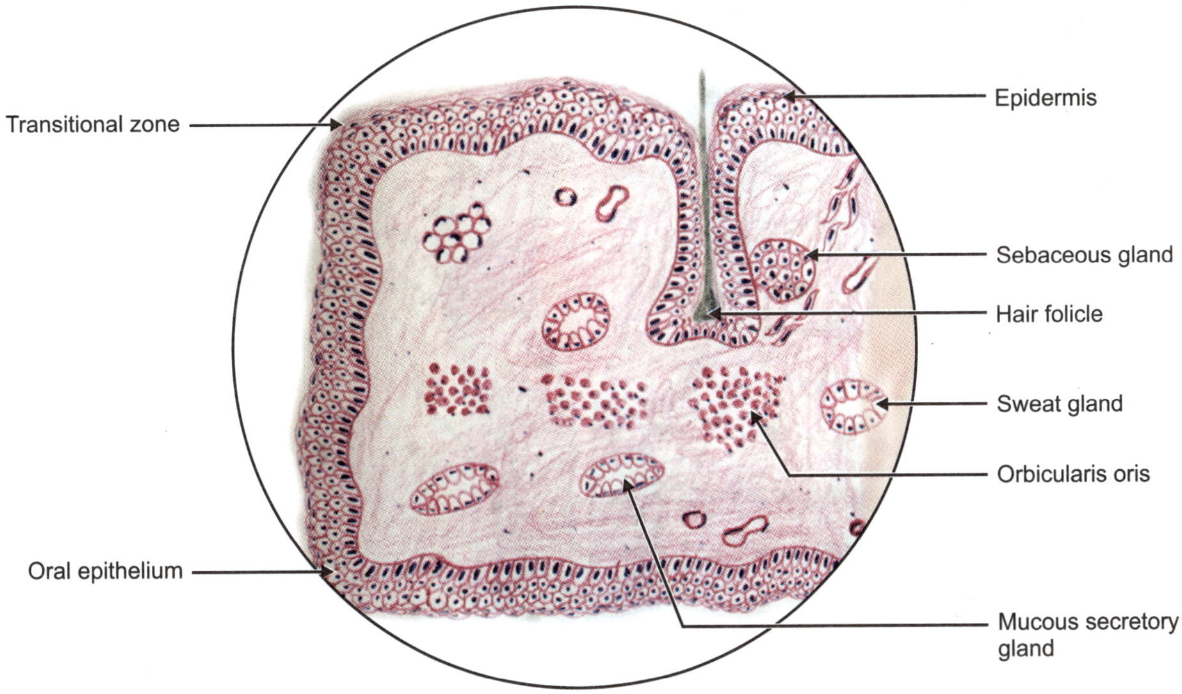
Epidermis
Transitional zone
Sebaceous gland
Hair folicle
Sweat gland
Orbicularis oris
Oral epithelium
Mucous secretory
gland

TONGUE: FILIFORM AND FUNGIFORM PAPILLAE

Filiform papillae: They are numerous conical shaped projections present on the dorsal surface of the tongue. It is lined by stratified squamous non-keratinized epithelium except along its tips where it is keratinized (para keratinization).

These papillae do not have taste buds.

Fungiform papillae: Mushroom-shaped projections lined by stratified squamous non-keratinized epithelium distributed along the margins and tips of the tongue.

They have taste buds along their upper surface.

Both the papillae consist of core of lamina propria (connective tissue).

Beneath the mucous membrane the substance of the tongue consists of sections of skeletal muscle fibres and are arranged in various directions.

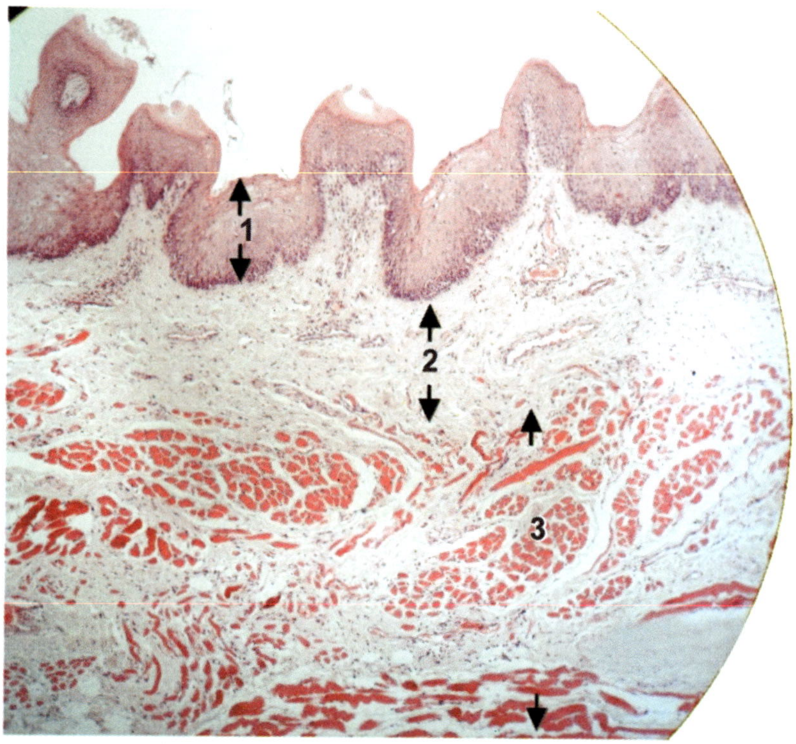

1. Stratified squamous non-keratinized epithelium
2. Lamina propria
3. Skeletal muscle

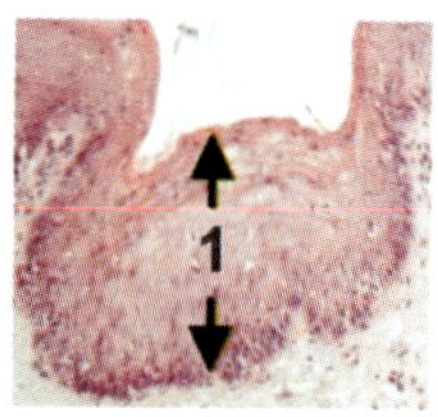

Key Features to Identify the Slide

- Conical-shaped filiform papillae lined by stratified squamous keratinized epithelium along its tips
- Mushroom-shaped fungiform papillae lined by stratified squamous non-keratinized epithelium
- Taste buds along the apical surface of the fungiform papillae
- Sections of skeletal muscle fibres forming the core of the tongue

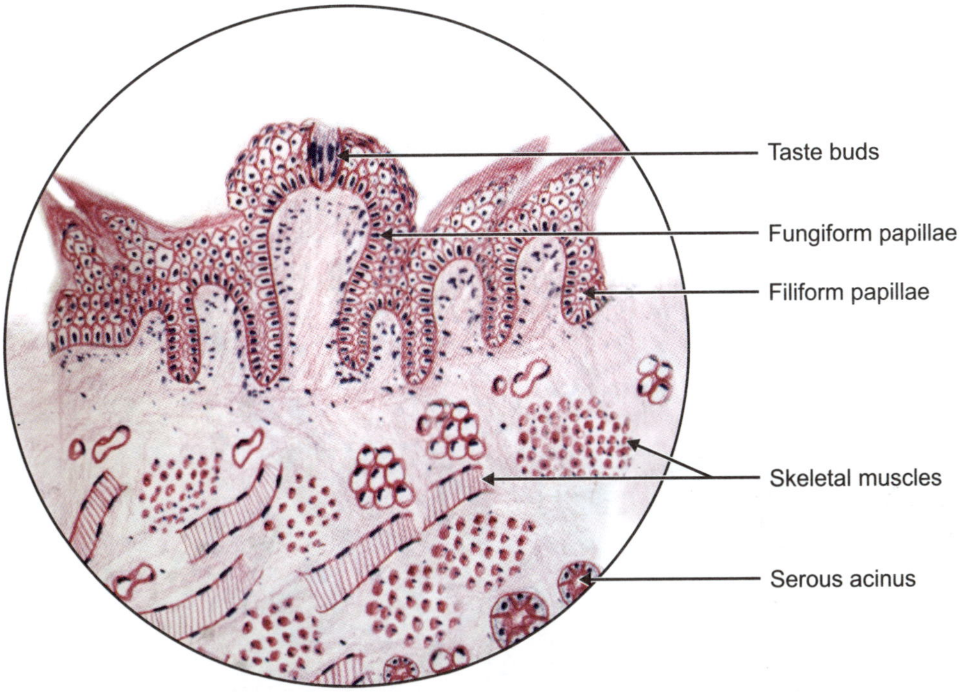
Taste buds
Fungiform papillae
Filiform papillae
Skeletal muscles
Serous acinus

TONGUE: CIRCUMVALLATE PAPILLA

These papillae are distributed anterior to sulcus terminalis.

The mucous membrane is lined by non-keratinized stratified squamous epithelium.

The papilla is surrounded by circular sulcus (trench) and the wall of the sulcus contains numerous taste buds.

The core of each papillae consists of connective tissue, blood vessels, nerves and lymphatics.

The region beneath the papilla consists of serous glands known as Von Ebner's gland the duct of which open into the base of the sulcus.

Taste buds: They are oval shaped, pale staining neurosensory epithelial structures embedded in the epithelium of the tongue. The cells are elongated and they converge towards surface depression called taste pore.

Histologically they are made up of sensory/neuroepithelial cells, supporting cells and basal cells.

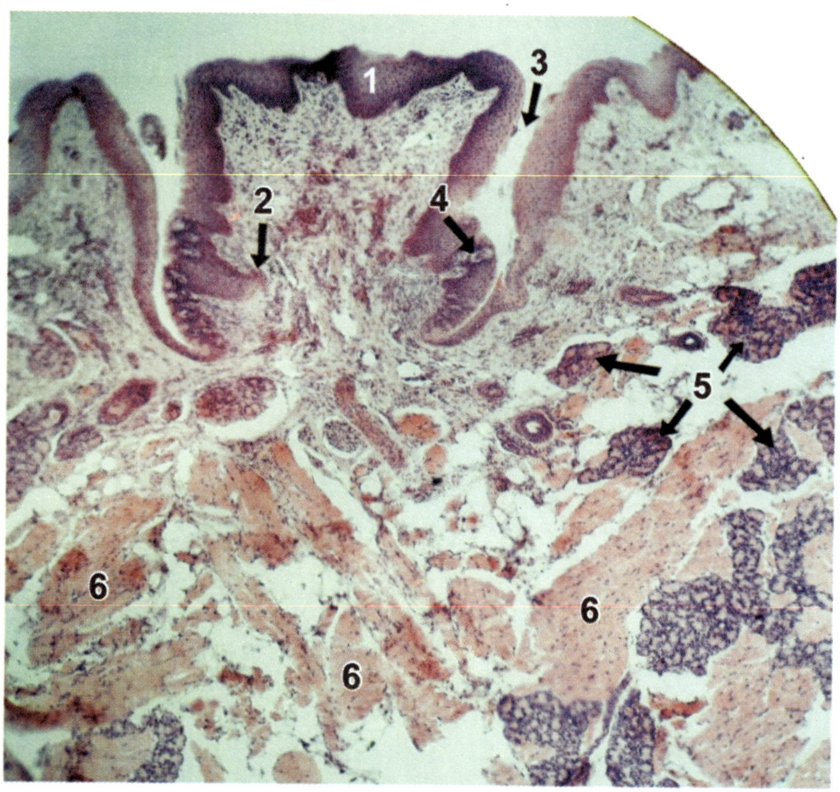

1. Stratified squamous non-keratinized epithelium
2. Secondary papillation
3. Furrow (trench)
4. Taste buds (in the lateral wall)
5. Serous (Von Ebner's) glands (in lamina propria)
6. Skeletal muscle zone

Key Features to Identify the Slide

- Mucous membrane lined by stratified squamous non-keratinized epithelium
- Presence of numerous taste buds along the lateral wall of papillae
- Presence of Von Ebner's glands in lamina propria
- Sections of skeletal muscle fibres forming the core of the tongue

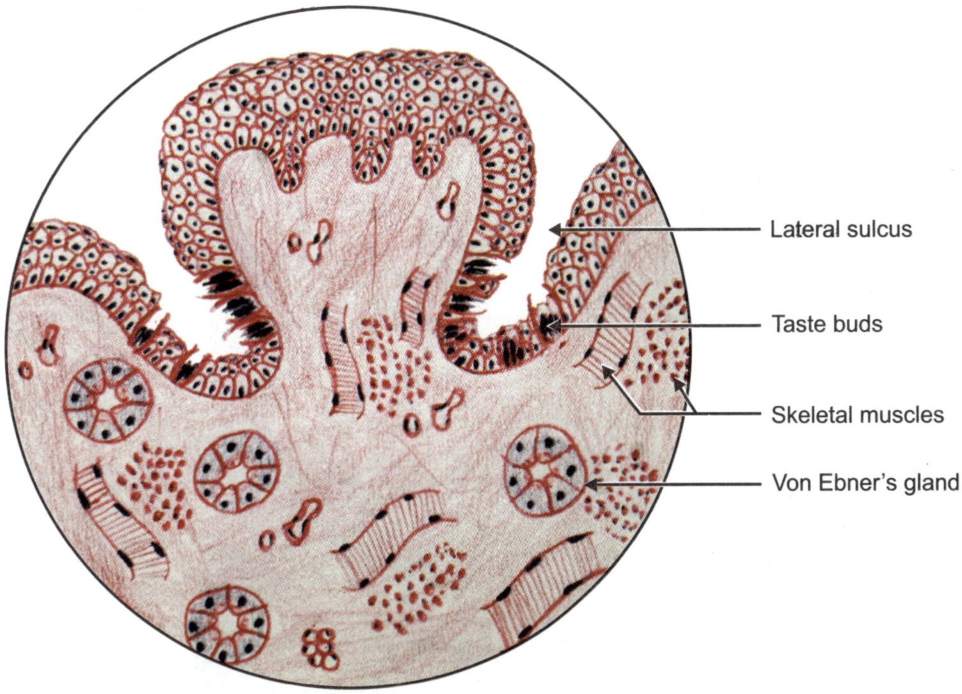
Lateral sulcus
Taste buds
Skeletal muscles
Von Ebner's gland

SEROUS SALIVARY GLAND

Connective tissue: Parotid gland is covered by capsule and septa extends from the capsule dividing the gland into lobes and lobules.

Serous acini: Lined by pyramidal cells with round nucleus towards the base of cell exhibits biphasic staining—eosinophilic in the apical part due to presence of zymogen granules, basophilic toward the base due to presence of large amount of rough endoplasmic reticulum.

- Acini shows narrow lumen.
- Each acinus is surrounded by myoepithelial cells that would help in expelling the secretion.

Ducts: Intralobular ducts are of two varieties: (a) Intercalated lined by low cuboidal epithelium that commences from the lumen of the acinus; (b) Striated duct—lined by simple columnar epithelium with basal infolding giving a striated appearance, it connects intercalated duct with interlobular duct.

- Also, sections of interlobular and lobar ducts are seen along the connective tissue septa.

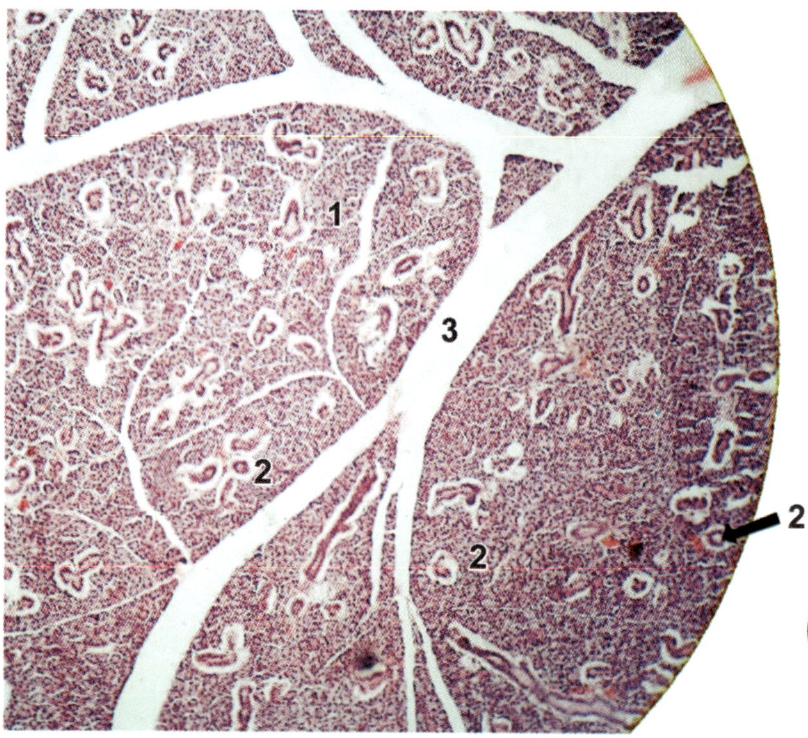

1. Serous acini (deep eosin stain)
2. Intralobular ducts
3. Interlobular connective tissue

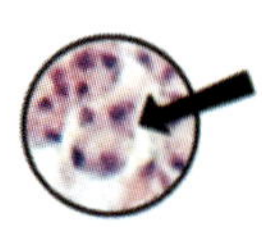

Key Features to Identify the Slide

- Presence of numerous serous acini with narrow lumen
- Pyramidal cells with biphasic staining
- Round nucleus more toward the base
- Numerous ducts are seen—interlobular and intralobular ducts

Example

- Parotid gland

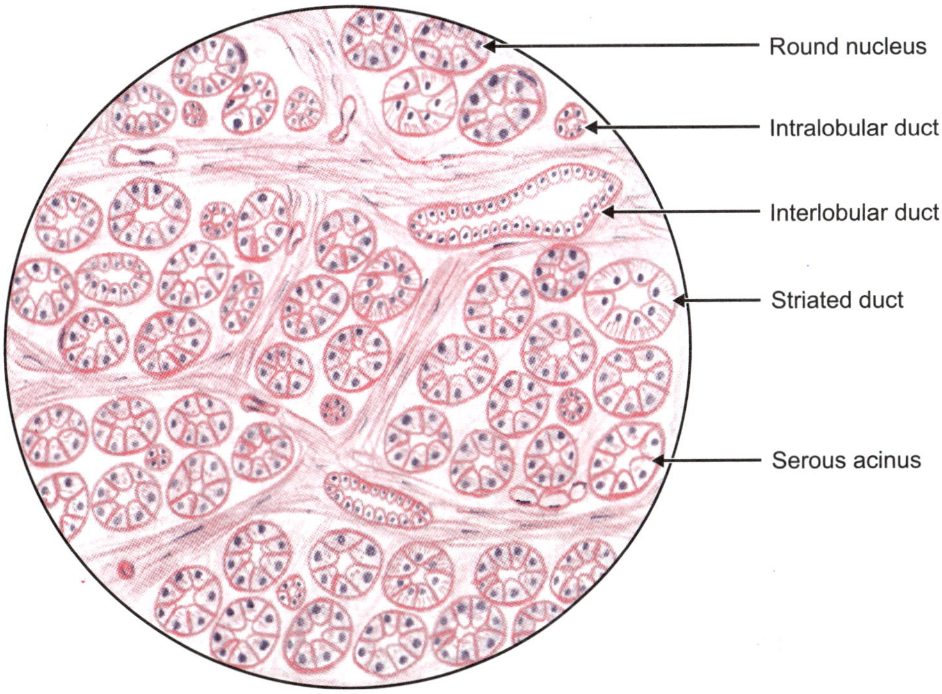
Round nucleus
Intralobular duct
Interlobular duct
Striated duct
Serous acinus

MUCOUS SALIVARY GLAND

In sublingual salivary gland capsule is not well defined.

Mucus acini: Lined by columnar/pyramidal cells with flat nucleus toward the base.

- Apical part of the cell has mucinogen granules giving vacuolated appearance to the cell.
- Each acinus exhibits wider lumen.

Ducts: Intralobular ducts are rarely seen.

- Sections of interlobular and lobar ducts are seen in the connective tissue septa

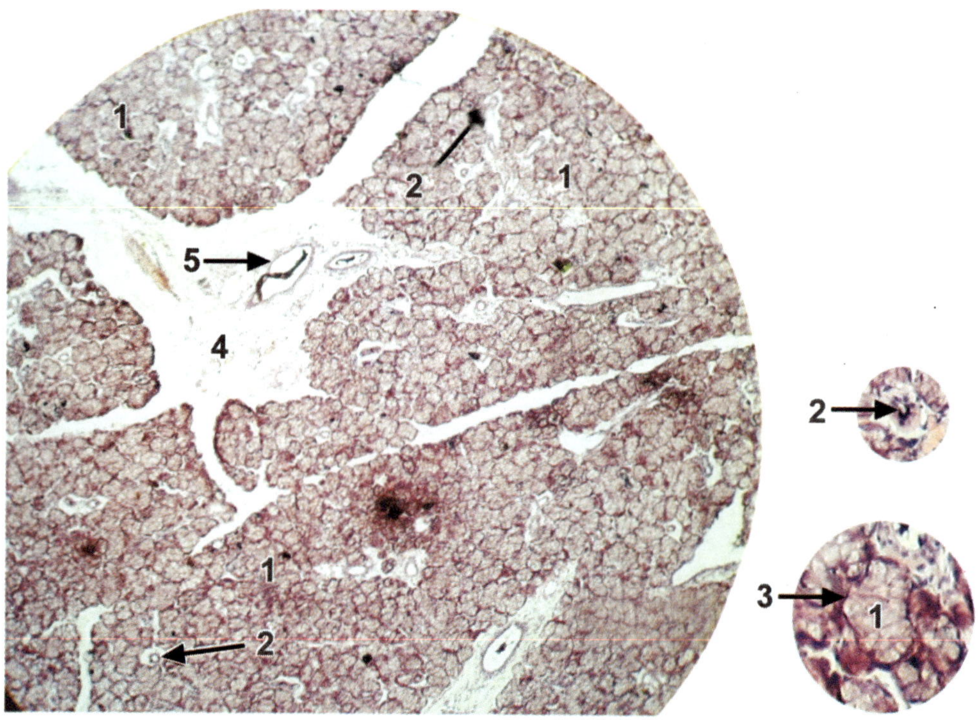

1. Mucous acini (pale stained)
2. Intralobular duct
3. Serous demilune
4. Interlobular connective tissue
5. Interlobular duct

Key Features to Identify the Slide

- Presence of numerous mucous acini with large lumen
- Flat nucleus at the base of each cell
- Numerous ducts are seen—interlobular and intralobular ducts

Example

- Sublingual salivary gland

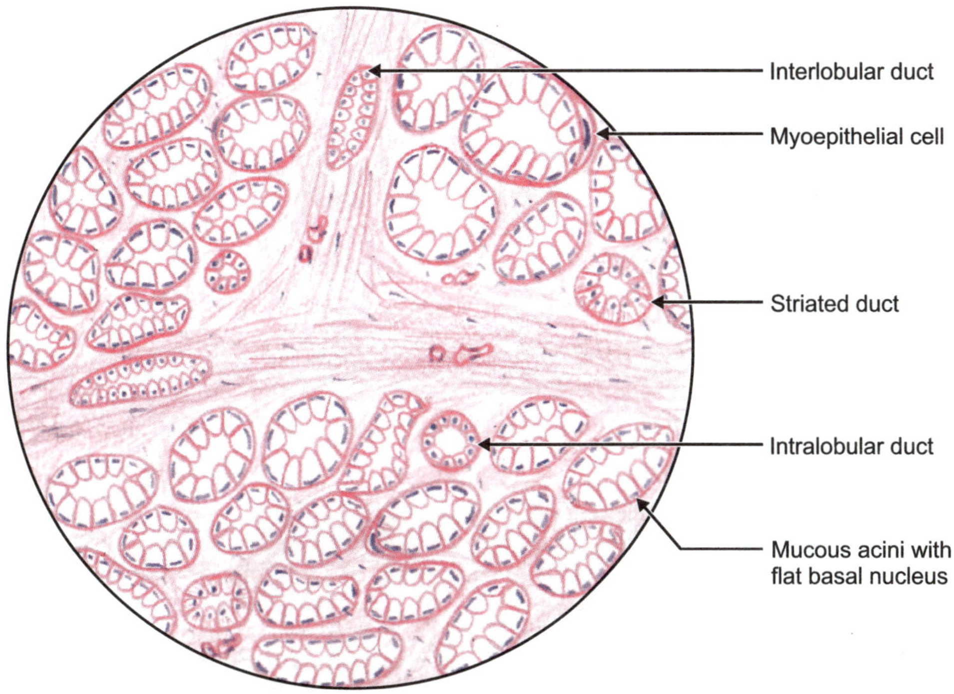
Interlobular duct
Myoepithelial cell
Striated duct
Intralobular duct
Mucous acini with
flat basal nucleus

MIXED SALIVARY GLAND

Connective tissue: Submandibular gland is covered by capsule and septa extends from the capsule dividing the gland into lobes and lobules.

Acini: Presence of both serous and mucous acini.

Serous demilunes: Mucus acini being capped by few serous cells.

- Appearance of serous demilunes are considered as histological artefacts due to chemical fixation.

Ducts: Intralobular ducts are of two varieties

(a) Intercalated duct—lined by low cuboidal epithelium that commences from the lumen of the acinus.

(b) Striated duct—lined by simple columnar epithelium with basal infolding giving a striated appearance, it connects intercalated duct with interlobular duct.

- Also, sections of interlobular and lobar ducts are seen along the connective tissue septa.

Applied Aspects of Oral Cavity and Associated Structures

1. Glossitis—inflammation of the tongue due to allergy, infection, injury and nutritional disorders.
2. Pleomorphic adenoma—most common benign tumor of parotid gland arising from ductal and myoepithelial cells.

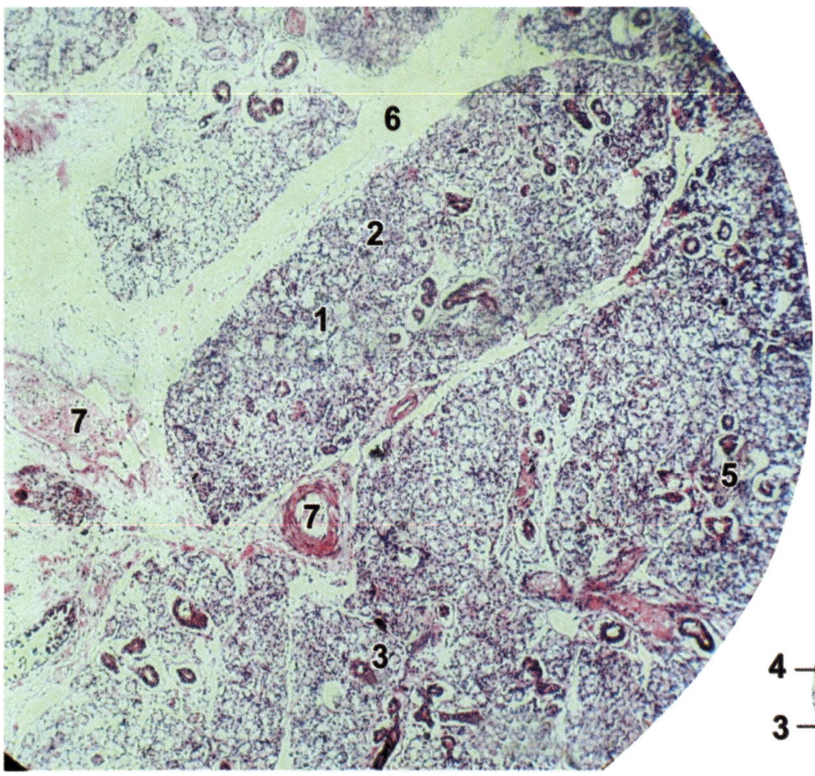

1. Mucous acini
2. Serous acini
3. Intercalated duct
4. Serous demilune
5. Intralobular ducts
6. Interlobular connective tissue
7. Blood vessels

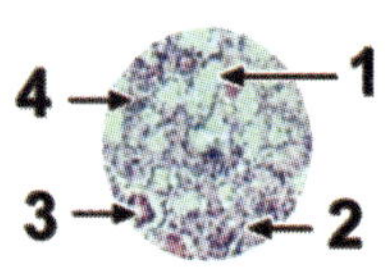

Key Features to Identify the Slide

- Presence of both serous and mucous acini
- Presence of serous demilunes over the mucous acini
- Numerous ducts are seen—interlobular and intralobular ducts

Example

– Submandibular salivary gland

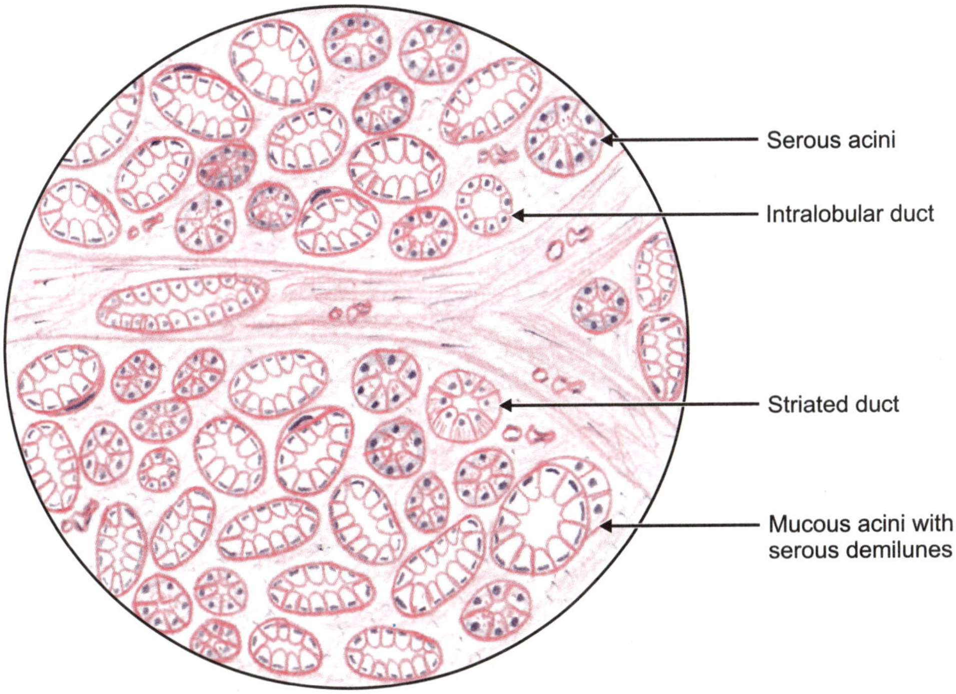
Serous acini
Intralobular duct
Striated duct
Mucous acini with
serous demilunes

QUESTIONS

1. What are Von Ebner's glands? 2M
2. Describe the serous demilunes. 2M
3. Microscopic anatomy of circumvallate papilla. 2M
4. Histology of parotid gland. 5M
5. What are myoepithelial cells. 2M
6. Name and describe the microscopic structure of submandibular salivary glands. 5M
7. Explain the layers of lip. 5M

Figures/Notes

12 Digestive System (AN 52.1)

OESOPHAGUS

Mucosa— consists of following layers:

(a) Epithelium—lined by non-keratinized stratified squamous epithelium.

(b) Lamina propria—made up of connective tissue containing scattered groups of lymphoid follicles, small tubular mucous glands are seen in this region.

(c) Muscularis mucosa composed mainly of longitudinal smooth muscle. It is thicker when compared to other parts of alimentary canal.

Submucosa: Consists of irregular dense connective tissue made up of elastic fibres, which are important in the reclosure of oesophageal lumen after peristaltic dilatation.

It also consists of blood vessels, nerves and tubuloalveolar mucous glands.

Muscularis externa: Consists of outer longitudinal and inner circular muscle layers.

In the upper 1/3rd of the oesophagus it is formed by skeletal muscle.

In the middle 1/3rd—by smooth muscle fascicles intermingled with striated muscle and in the lower 1/3rd—only smooth muscle is seen.

A well-formed myenteric plexus of nerve fibres are present between the two muscle layers.

Serosa/Adventitia consists of loose areolar connective tissue, except in the lowest 1 inch, where it is covered by serosa.

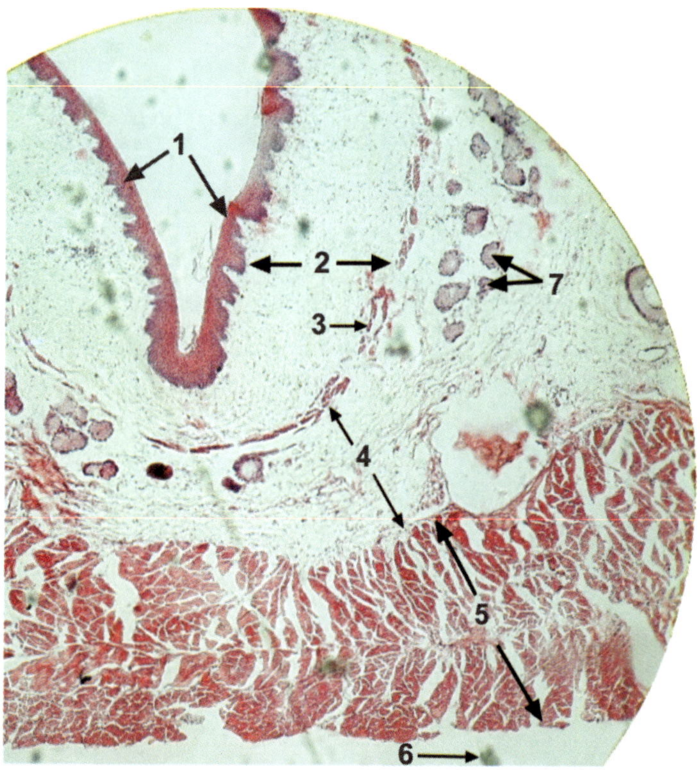

1. Stratified squamous non-keratinized epithelium
2. Lamina propria
3. Muscularis mucosae (smooth muscle)
4. Submucosa
5. Muscularis externa
6. Adventitia
7. Oesophageal glands (mucous) in submucosa

MUCOSA

Key Features to Identify the Slide

- Mucous membrane lined by stratified squamous non-keratinized epithelium
- Oesophageal glands in submucosa
- Muscularis externa showing inner circular and outer longitudinal muscle layers

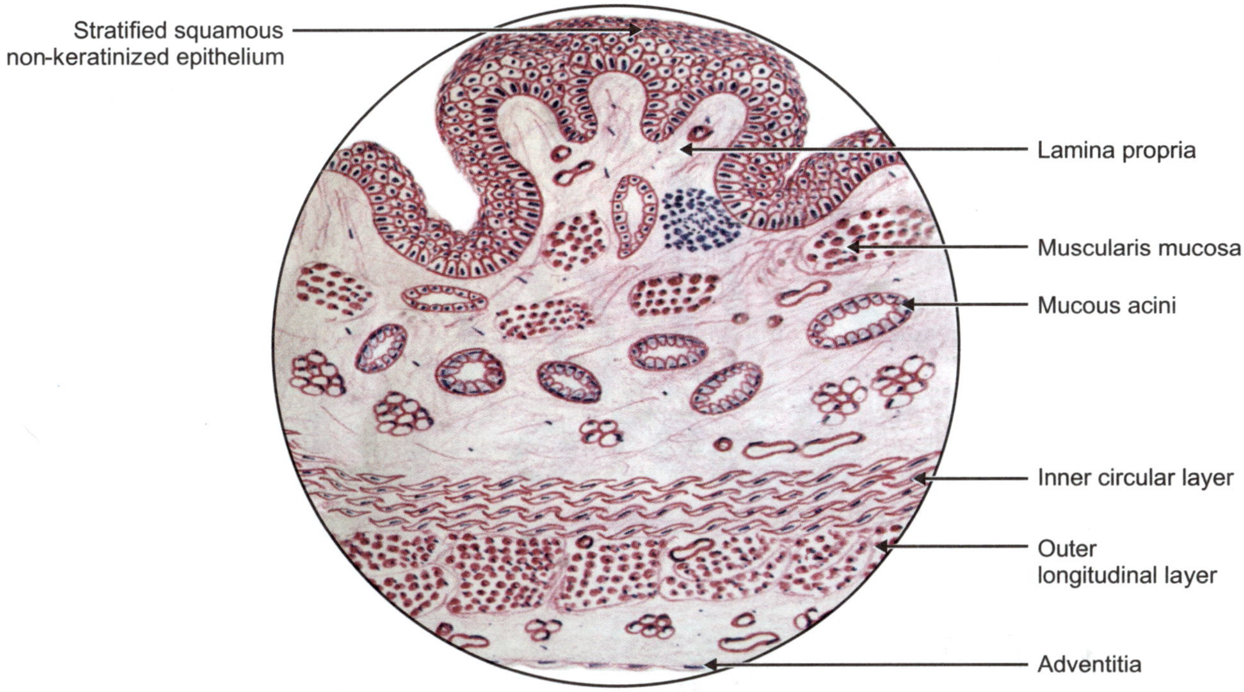
Stratified squamous
non-keratinized epithelium
Lamina propria
Muscularis mucosa
Mucous acini
Inner circular layer
Outer
longitudinal layer
Adventitia

STOMACH: FUNDUS

Mucosa consists of:

(a) Epithelium—made up of simple columnar epithelium lining the short gastric pits. The cells are involved in secretion of mucus which forms a thick protective and lubricant layer over the surface.

(b) Lamina propria—simple tubular glands are present which extend from gastric pit to the muscularis mucosae. The wall of the gland is made up of five distinct cell types.

1. Chief cell—basal in position and secrete zymogen granules, hence they are basophilic.
2. Parietal cell (oxyntic cell): They are seen in apical half of the gland and secrete HCl and intrinsic factor hence they are eosinophilic.
3. Mucus neck cell—situated at the neck of the gland they are mucus secreting.
4. Stem cells
5. Enteroendocrine cell

(c) Muscularis mucosae—made up of thin layer of smooth muscle arranged as inner circular and outer longitudinal layers.

Submucosa: It is a layer of loose connective tissue containing blood vessels and nerve plexus (Meissner's plexus).

Muscularis externa: It is a thick muscle coat arranged as innermost oblique, middle circular and outer longitudinal layers of smooth muscle fibres, in between them myenteric plexus or Auerbach's plexus of nerve fibres are seen.

Serosa / Adventitia: Visceral peritoneum made up of a layer of loose connective tissue covered by mesothelium.

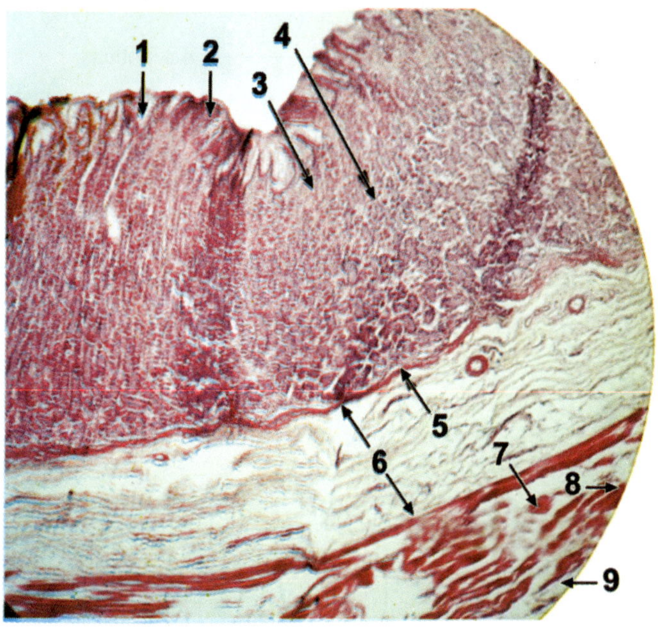

1. Gastric pits (shallow)
2. Epithelium (simple columnar)
3. Parietal cells
4. Chief cells
5. Muscularis mucosae
6. Submucosa
7. Inner circular
8. Outer longitudinal
9. Serosa

(3 and 4: Gastric glands in lamina propria; 7 and 8: Muscularis externa)

Key Features to Identify the Slide

- Mucous membrane lined by simple columnar epithelium
- Short gastric pits are present
- Presence of chief and parietal cells lining long gastric glands in lamina propria

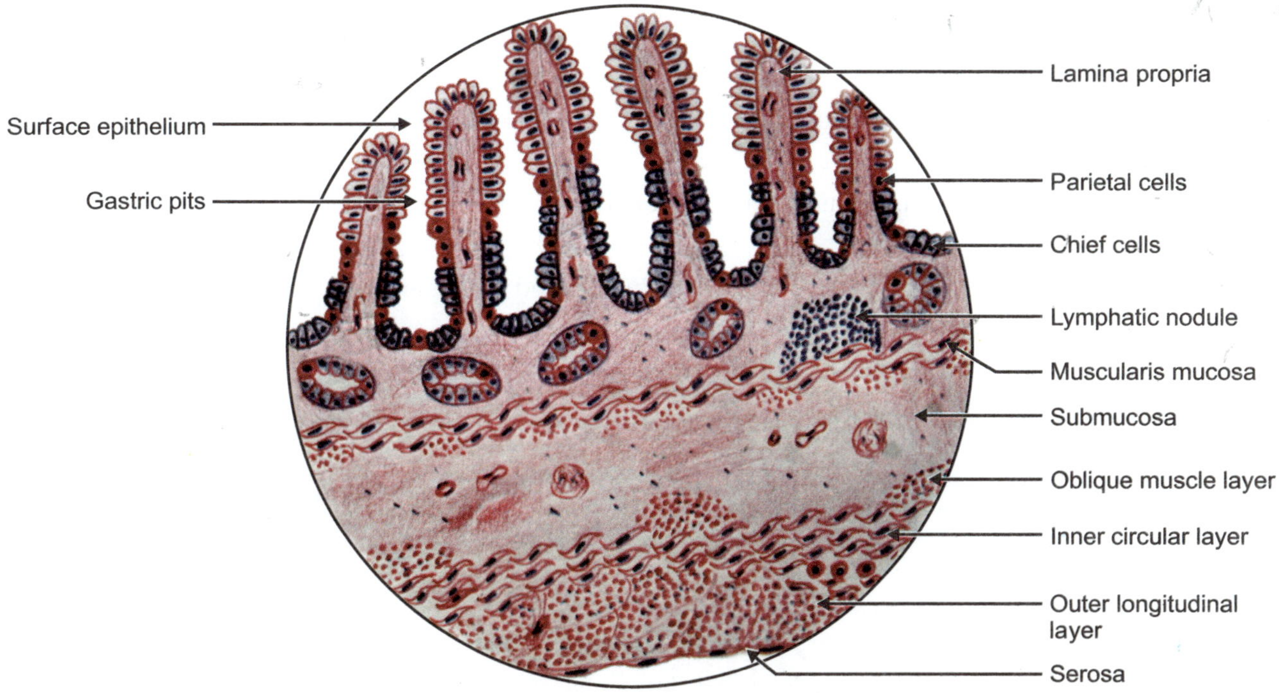
Surface epithelium
Gastric pits
Lamina propria
Parietal cells
Chief cells
Lymphatic nodule
Muscularis mucosa
Submucosa
Oblique muscle layer
Inner circular layer
Outer longitudinal layer
Serosa

STOMACH: PYLORUS

Mucosa consists of:

(a) Epithelium—made up of simple columnar mucous secreting epithelium lining the gastric pits which are deep occupying about 2/3rd of mucosal depth.

The glands are short and convoluted.

(b) Lamina propria: The glands are predominantly lined by mucus secreting cells. Enteroendocrine cells are also present in this region.

(c) Muscularis mucosae—made up of thin layer of smooth muscle arranged as inner circular and outer longitudinal layers.

Submucosa—it is a layer of loose connective tissue containing blood vessels and nerve plexus (Meissner's plexus).

Muscularis externa—it is a thick muscle coat arranged as innermost oblique, middle circular and outer longitudinal layers of smooth muscle fibres. In between them myenteric plexus or Auerbach's plexus of nerve fibres are seen.

Serosa / Adventitia—visceral peritoneum made up of a layer of loose connective tissue covered by mesothelium.

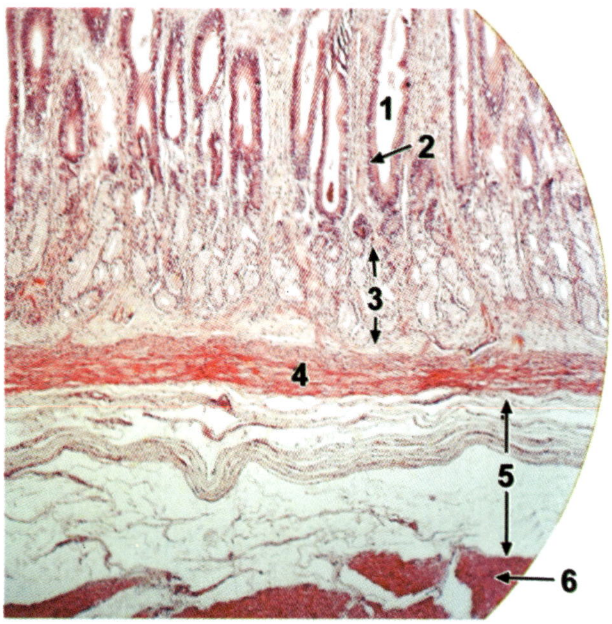

1. Gastric pits (deeper and wider)
2. Epithelium (simple columnar)
3. Pyloric glands in lamina propria
4. Muscularis mucosae
5. Submucosa
6. Muscularis externa

MUCOSA

Key Features to Identify the Slide

- Mucous membrane lined by simple columnar epithelium
- Presence of deep gastric pits
- Short pyloric glands present in lamina propria

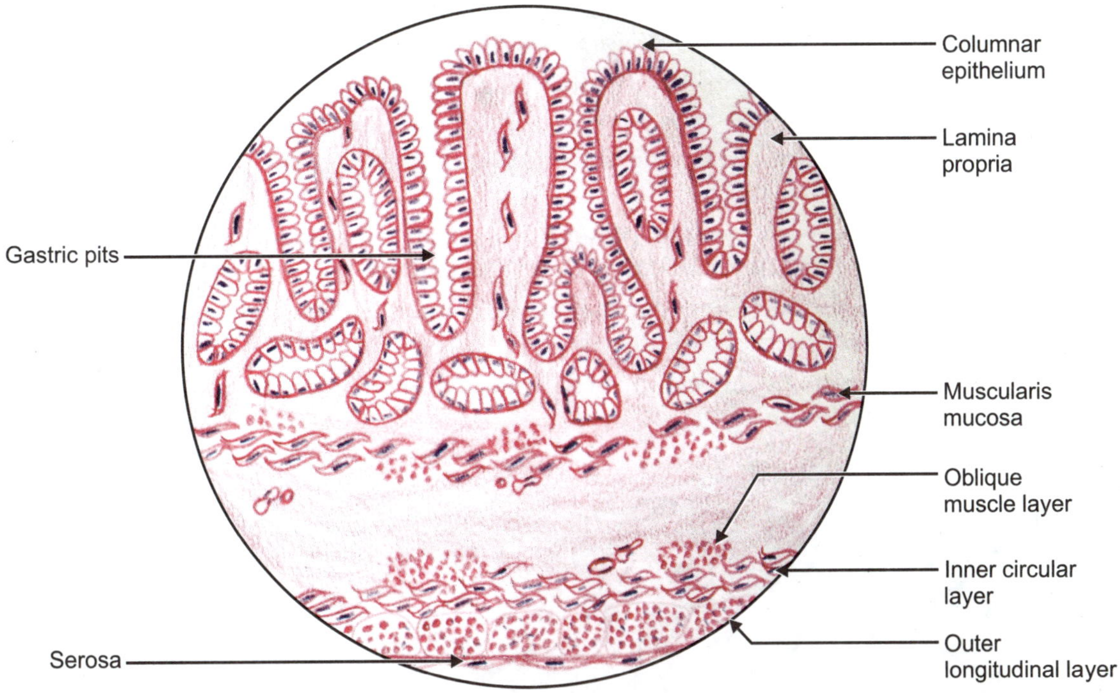
Columnar epithelium
Lamina propria
Gastric pits
Muscularis mucosa
Oblique muscle layer
Inner circular layer
Outer longitudinal layer
Serosa

DUODENUM

Mucosa: Shows finger like projections called villi lined by columnar epithelium with microvilli (striated border). Few goblet cells are seen between them.

- The core of the villus consists of loose connective tissue of lamina propria with capillaries, smooth muscles fibres and lymphatics (lacteals).

Lamina propria: Presence of intestinal glands (crypt of Lieberkühn) lined by columnar cells, goblet cells, Paneth cells and enteroendocrine cells and stem cells.

Muscularis mucosa: Consists of smooth muscle fibres arranged in inner circular and outer longitudinal layers. It sends fibres towards the core of the villi.

Submucosa: Completely filled with small branched tubuloacinar submucosal glands (Brunner's gland) which secretes alkaline mucus that neutralizes acid secreted from the stomach.

Muscularis externa: Made up of thick inner circular and thin outer longitudinal muscle layers. In between them myenteric (Auerbach's) plexus of nerve fibres are seen.

Serosa / Adventitia: Visceral peritoneum made up of a layer of loose connective tissue covered by mesothelium. The retroperitoneal part is covered by adventitia.

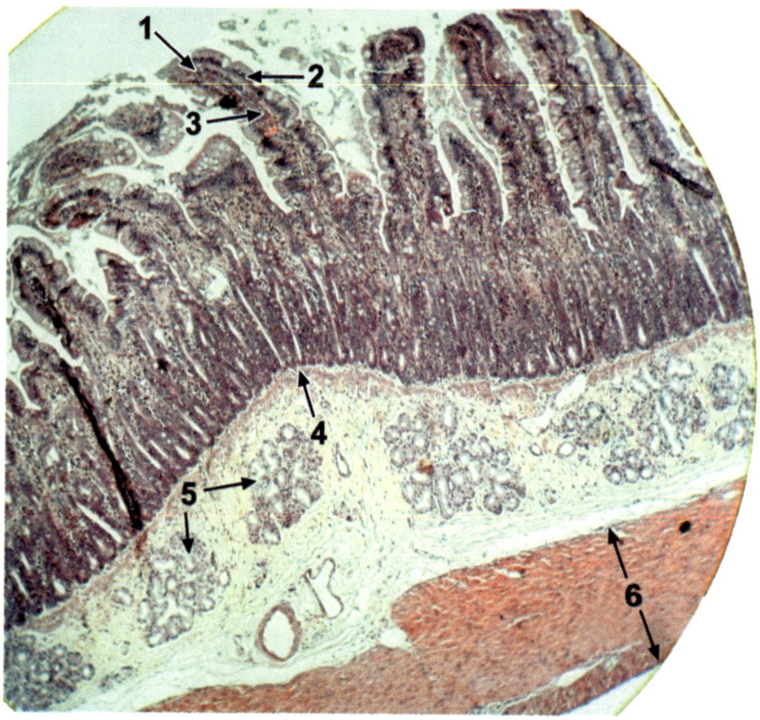

1. Villus
2. Simple columnar epithelium with striated border
3. Lamina propria
4. Muscularis mucosae
5. Brunner's gland in submucosa
6. Muscularis externa

MUCOSA

VILLUS

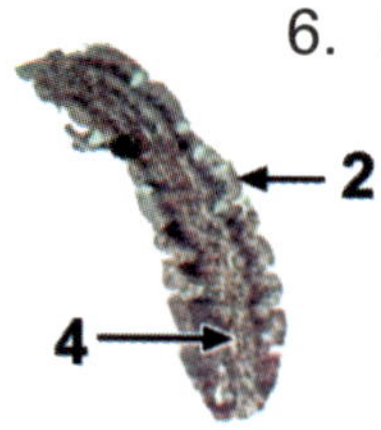

Key Features to Identify the Slide

- Presence of villi lined by simple columnar epithelium with microvilli [striated border]
- Presence of crypts of Lieberkühn
- Brunner's glands in submucosa

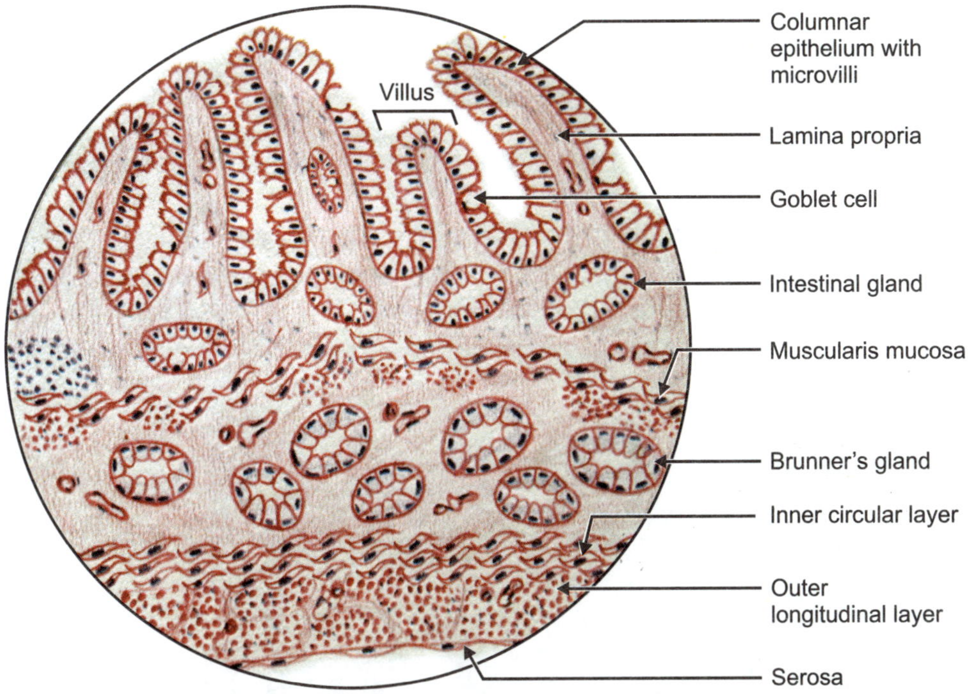
Villus
Columnar epithelium with microvilli
Lamina propria
Goblet cell
Intestinal gland
Muscularis mucosa
Brunner's gland
Inner circular layer
Outer longitudinal layer
Serosa

JEJUNUM

Mucosa: Shows large tongue shaped villi of different heights lined by columnar epithelium with microvilli (striated border). Few goblet cells are seen between them.

- The core of the villus consists of loose connective tissue of lamina propria with capillaries, smooth muscle fibres and lymphatics (lacteals).

Lamina propria: Presence of intestinal glands (crypt of Lieberkühn) lined by columnar cells, goblet cells, Paneth cells, enteroendocrine cells and stem cells.

Muscularis mucosa: Consists of smooth muscle fibres are arranged in inner circular and outer longitudinal layers. It sends fibres towards the core of the villi.

Submucosa: Made up of connective tissue, blood vessels, nerve plexus (Meissner's plexus) and lymphatics.

Muscularis externa: Made up of thick inner circular and thin outer longitudinal muscle layers. In between them myenteric (Auerbach's) plexus of nerve fibres are seen.

Serosa: Visceral peritoneum made up of a layer of loose connective tissue covered by mesothelium.

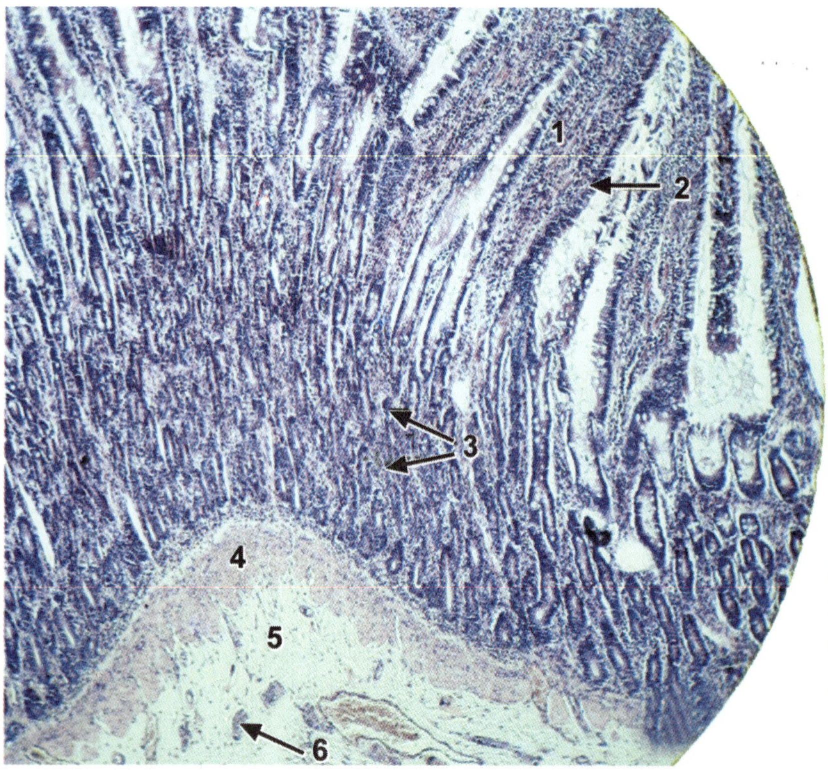

1. Villus
2. Simple columnar epithelium with striated border
3. Crypts of Lieberkühn extending into lamina propria
4. Muscularis mucosae
5. Submucosa
6. Muscularis externa

MUCOSA

VILLUS

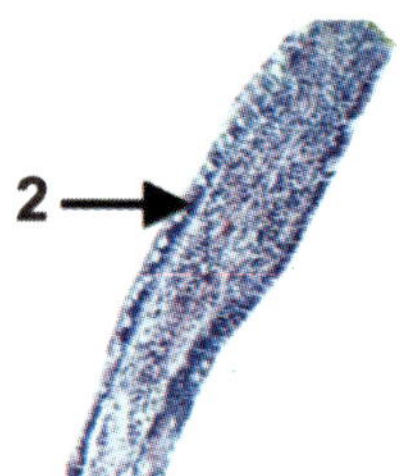

Key Features to Identify the Slide

- Numerous tongue-shaped villi lined by simple columnar epithelium with microvilli [striated border]
- Presence of goblet cells
- Presence of crypts of Lieberkühn (intestinal glands)

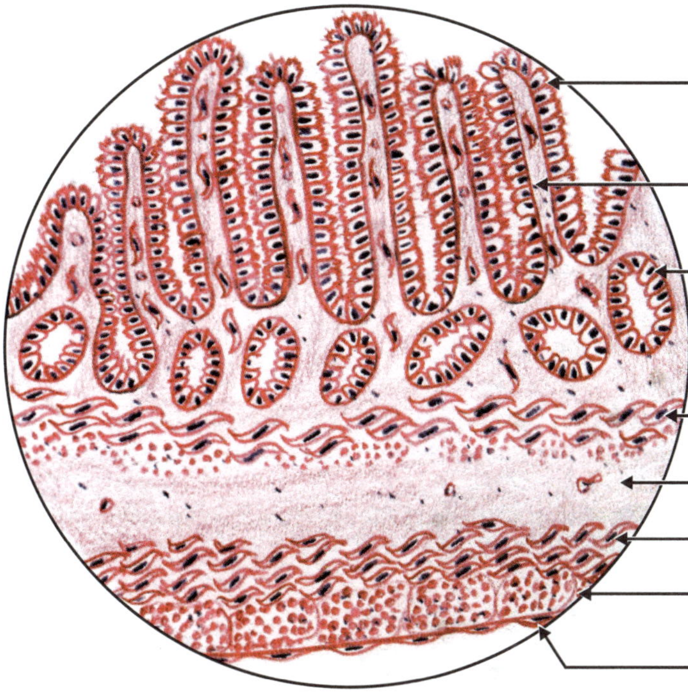
Simple columnar epithelium with microvilli
Lamina propria
Intestinal glands
Muscularis mucosa
Submucosa
Inner circular layer
Outer longitudinal layer
Serosa

ILEUM

Mucosa: Shows few short finger-shaped villi. Lined by columnar epithelium with microvilli (striated border). Numerous goblet cells are seen.

Lamina propria: Consists of aggregation of lymphoid follicles (Peyer's patches) which belong to MALT. Some of them develop germinal centre after exposure to antigen.

- The intestinal epithelium overlying these follicles consists of M-cells (microfold cells) in between the columnar cells.
- M-cells are considered as antigen presenting cells.

Submucosa: Made up of connective tissue, blood vessels, nerve plexus (Meissner's plexus) and lymphatics.

Muscularis externa—made up of thick inner circular and thin outer longitudinal muscle layers. In between them myenteric (Auerbach's) plexus of nerve fibres are seen.

Serosa: Visceral peritoneum made up of a layer of loose connective tissue covered by mesothelium.

Cells of intestinal glands:

1. Columnar cells/enterocytes—absorptive in nature.
2. Goblet cells—secrete mucus which provide lubrication.
3. Paneth cells—they contain acidophilic granules which secrete lysosome and antibacterial enzyme.
4. Enteroendocrine cells (APUD)—seen in the deeper parts of the gland, they secrete gastrin, somatostatin and histamine.
5. Stem cells—situated in the isthmus of the gland they are undifferentiated mitotic cells from which the other types of cells lining the gland are derived.

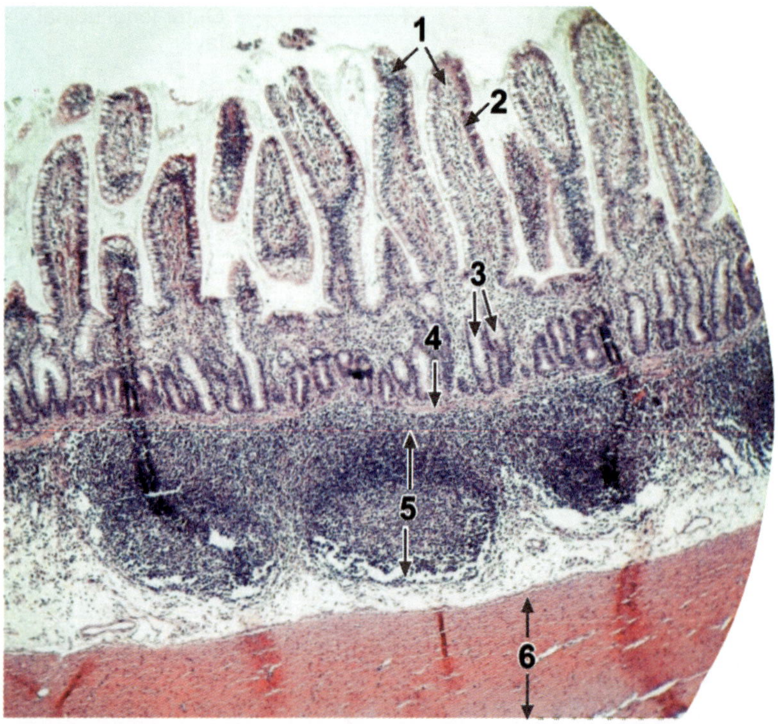

1. Villus
2. Simple columnar epithelium with striated border
3. Intestinal glands (crypts of Lieberkühn) extending into lamina propria
4. Muscularis mucosae
5. Peyer's patches (originate in lamina propria and extend into submucosa)
6. Muscularis externa

M U C O S A

Key Features to Identify the Slide

- Finger-shaped villi lined by simple columnar epithelium with microvilli [striated border]
- Presence of numerous goblet cells
- Peyer's patches [aggregated lymphoid follicles] seen in mucosa

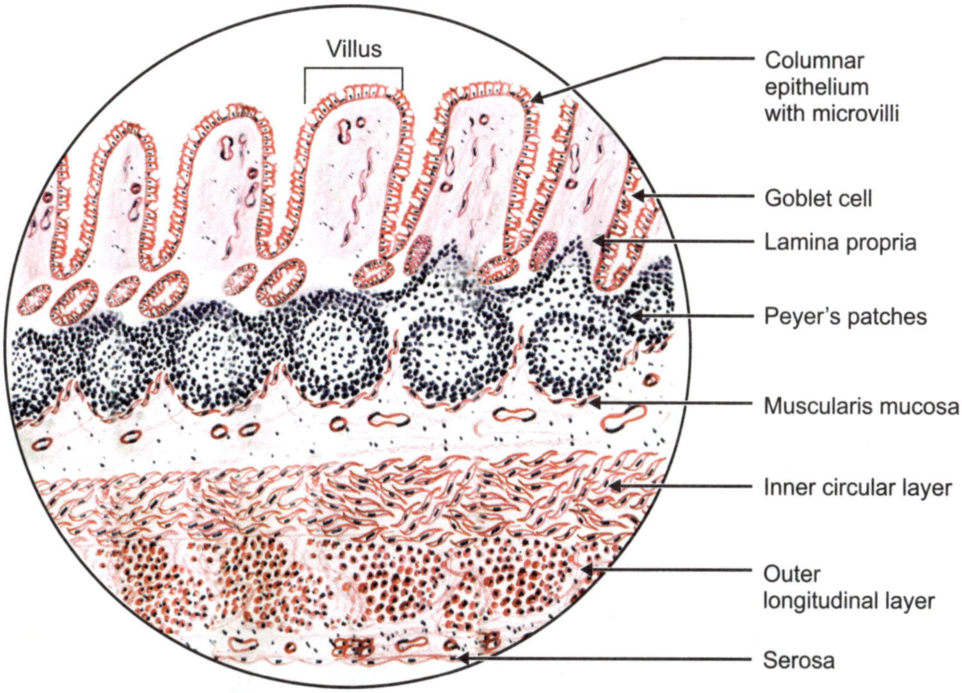
Villus
Columnar epithelium with microvilli
Goblet cell
Lamina propria
Peyer's patches
Muscularis mucosa
Inner circular layer
Outer longitudinal layer
Serosa

VERMIFORM APPENDIX

Mucosa: Lined by simple columnar epithelium with more number of goblet cells in between them.

Lamina propria: Is occupied with many lymphatic nodules and some exhibiting germinal centre.

- The epithelium lining the mucosal lymphoid tissue contains M-cells.
- Also contains few short intestinal glands (crypts)

Muscularis mucosa: Is present, as seen in the other region of small intestine, it is disrupted at places where lymphatic nodules extend into submucosa.

Submucosa: Made up of connective tissue, blood vessels, nerve plexus (Meissner's plexus) and lymphatics.

- It may show extension of lymphatic nodules.

Muscularis externa: Made up of thick inner circular and thin outer longitudinal muscle layers. In between them myenteric (Auerbach's) plexus of nerve fibres are seen.

Serosa: Visceral peritoneum made up of a layer of loose connective tissue covered by mesothelium.

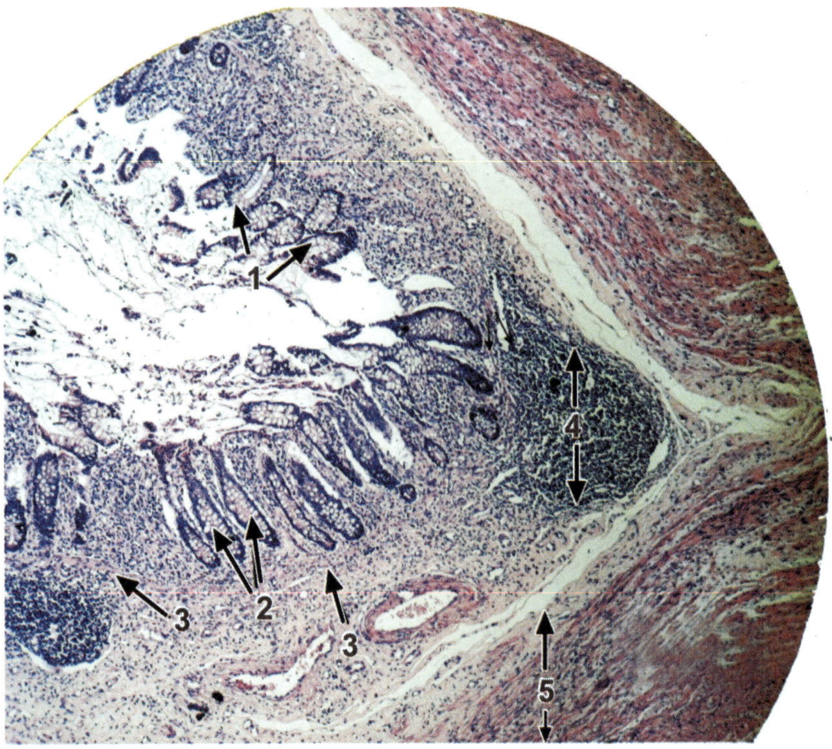

1. Simple columnar epithelium with numerous goblet cells
2. Intestinal glands (crypts of Lieberkühn) into lamina propria
3. Muscularis mucosae
4. Lymphatic nodule (originate in lamina propria and extend into submucosa)
5. Muscularis externa

M U C O S A

Key Features to Identify the Slide

- Absence of villi
- Mucosa lined by simple columnar epithelium with more number of goblet cells
- Aggregation of lymphoid follicles in lamina propria
- Absence of taenia coli

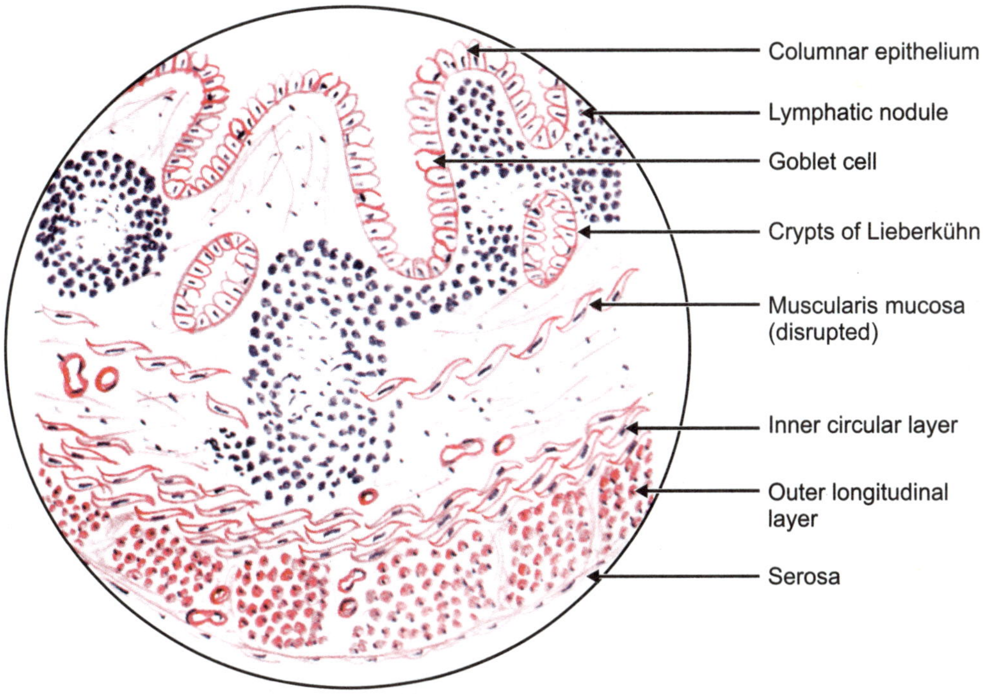
Columnar epithelium
Lymphatic nodule
Goblet cell
Crypts of Lieberkühn
Muscularis mucosa (disrupted)
Inner circular layer
Outer longitudinal layer
Serosa

LARGE INTESTINE/COLON

Mucosa: Lined by simple columnar epithelium with more number of goblet cells in between them. Mucosal folds and villi are absent.

Lamina propria: Is occupied with tubular glands (crypts). The glands are straight and longer when compared to the small intestine. The glands are lined by columnar cells, goblet cells, neuroendocrine cells and stem cells. Paneth cells are occasionally seen (in caecum only).

Muscularis mucosa: Is present, as seen in the other region of small intestine.

Submucosa: Made up of connective tissue, blood vessels, nerve plexus (Meissner's plexus) and lymphatics.

Muscularis externa: Inner circular and outer longitudinal muscle layers are seen. The logitudinal muscle layer is arranged into three thick bands called taenia coli.

Serosa / Adventitia: Visceral peritoneum made up of a layer of loose connective tissue covered by mesothelium. The retroperitoneal part is covered by adventitia.

Applied Aspects of Digestive System

1. Barrett's oesophagus: In the lower end of oesophagus the squamous epithelium is replaced by columnar epithelium due to gastro-oesophageal reflux disease (GERD).
2. Ulcerative colitis—inflammation of colon and rectum involving the mucosa and submucosal layers.

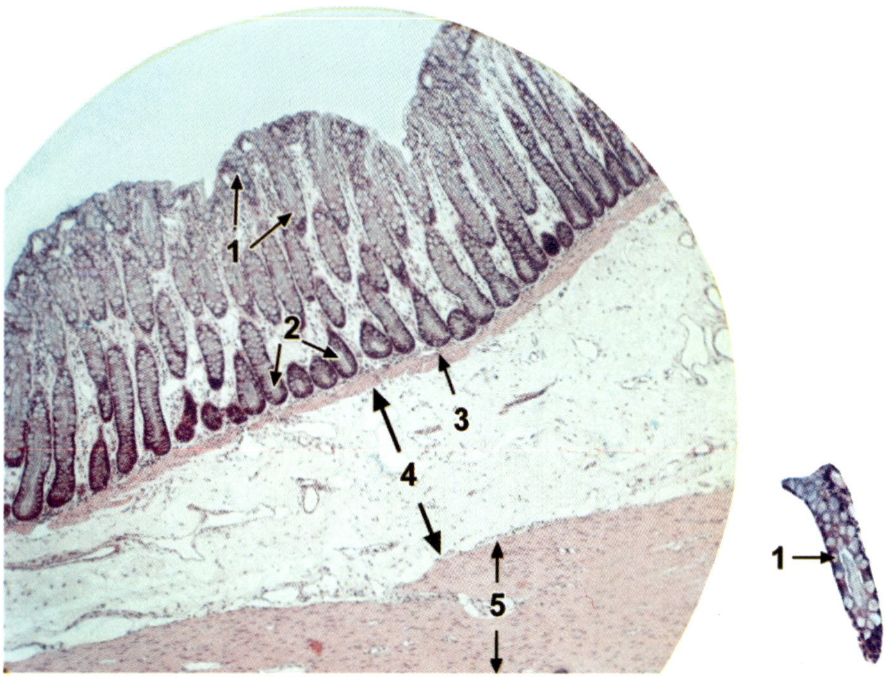

1. Simple columnar epithelium with plenty of goblet cells
2. Intestinal glands (crypts of Lieberkühn) in lamina propria
3. Muscularis mucosae
4. Submucosa
5. Muscularis externa (taenia coli)

M U C O S A

Key Features to Identify the Slide

- Lined by simple columnar epithelium with more number of goblet cells
- Villi are absent
- Taenia coli in muscularis externa

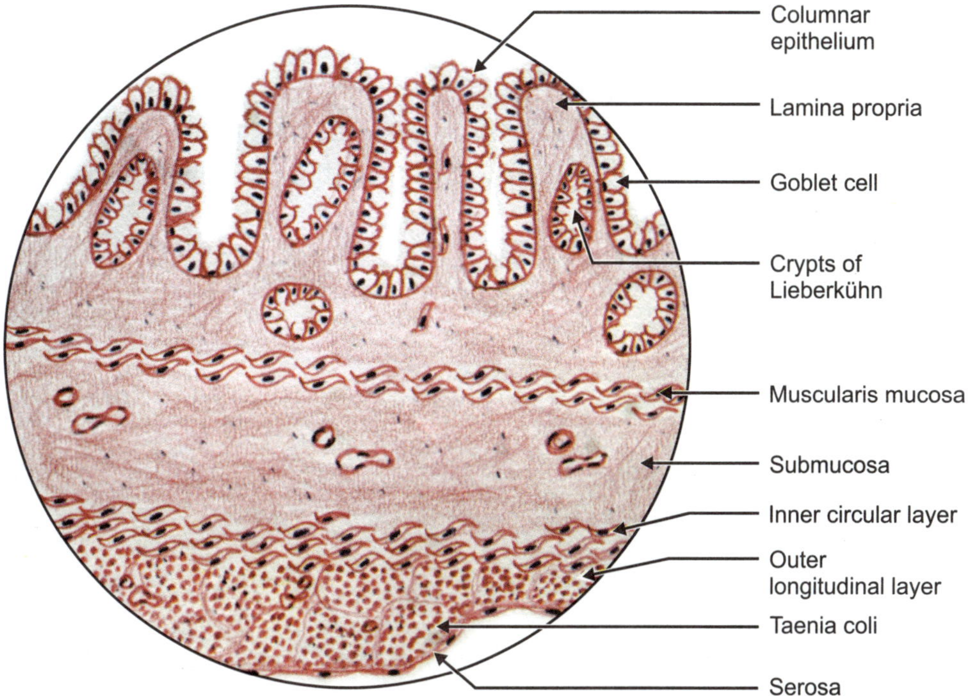
Columnar epithelium
Lamina propria
Goblet cell
Crypts of Lieberkühn
Muscularis mucosa
Submucosa
Inner circular layer
Outer longitudinal layer
Taenia coli
Serosa

QUESTIONS

1. What are the layers you observe under a microscope when looking at the gastrointestinal tract? 2M
2. Define gastric glands, including their parts, types of cells, and the differences between those in the fundus and pylorus. 5M
3. Explain the microscopic changes that occur at the cardio-oesophageal junction. 5M
4. Compare the microscopic features of the duodenum, jejunum, and ileum. 5M
5. Enumerate the types of cells found in gastric glands and elaborate on their functions. 5M
6. How do the crypts of Lieberkühn in the small intestine differ from those in the large intestine? 2M
7. What are Peyer's patches. 2M
8. Write the name and location of the nerve plexus present in GIT. 2M

Figures/Notes

LIVER

Stroma: Consists of connective tissue capsule (Glisson's capsule).

- At the hilum connective tissue enters the parenchyma of the gland giving rise to septae and trabeculae dividing the parenchyma into lobules. Connective tissue carries blood vessels and ducts along the trabeculae.

Parenchyma: Hexagonal lobules form structural and functional unit of the liver.

At the corners of each lobule are small triangular areas of connective tissue containing branches of portal vein, hepatic artery and interlobular bile duct.

- In the centre of each lobule is the central vein.
- Radiating from the central vein are hepatocytes arranged in one or two cells thick plate. These cells are separated by hepatic sinusoids.

The sinusoids are lined by endothelial cells and phagocytic cells called Kupffer's cells.

- In the interface between an adjacent pair of liver cells in a plate there exists bile canaliculi which drains the bile towards the portal triad.

Portal lobule: It is triangular in shape with portal triad in the centre and the central vein at each corner.

Hepatic acinus: At the opposite angles are central veins and at the other two opposite angles are the portal triads.

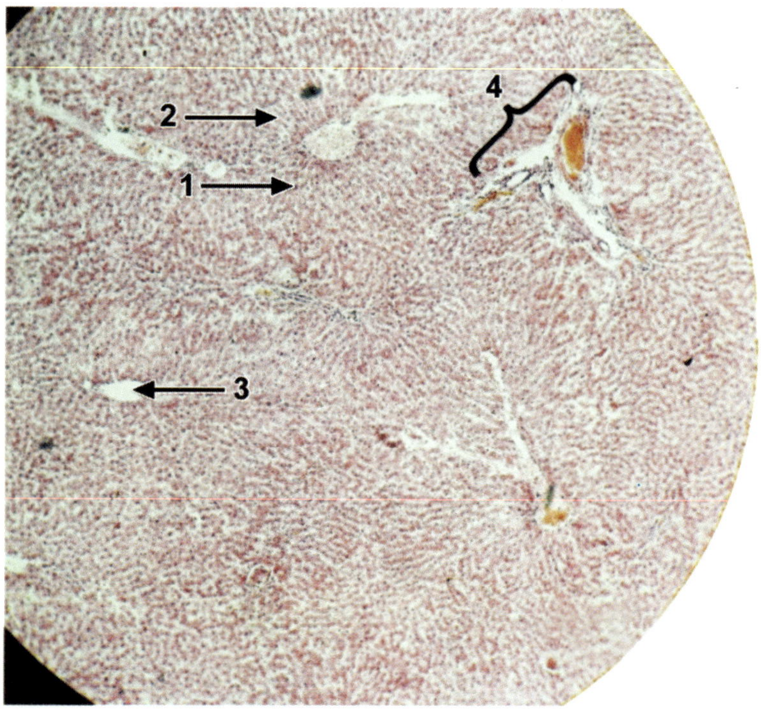

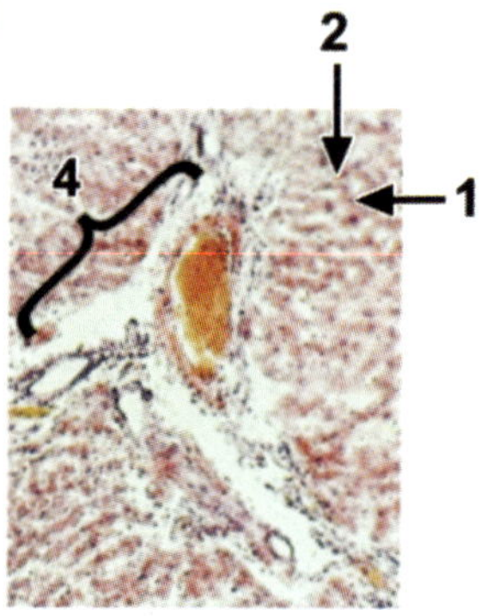

1. Radiating plates of hepatic cells
2. Hepatic sinusoid
3. Central vein
4. Portal triad containing interlobular branches of
   - Portal vein
   - Bile duct
   - Hepatic artery

Key Features to Identify the Slide

- Presence of hexagonal hepatic lobules
- Radiating cords of hepatocytes from the central vein
- Portal triads containing branches of hepatic artery, portal vein and bile duct at the periphery of each lobule

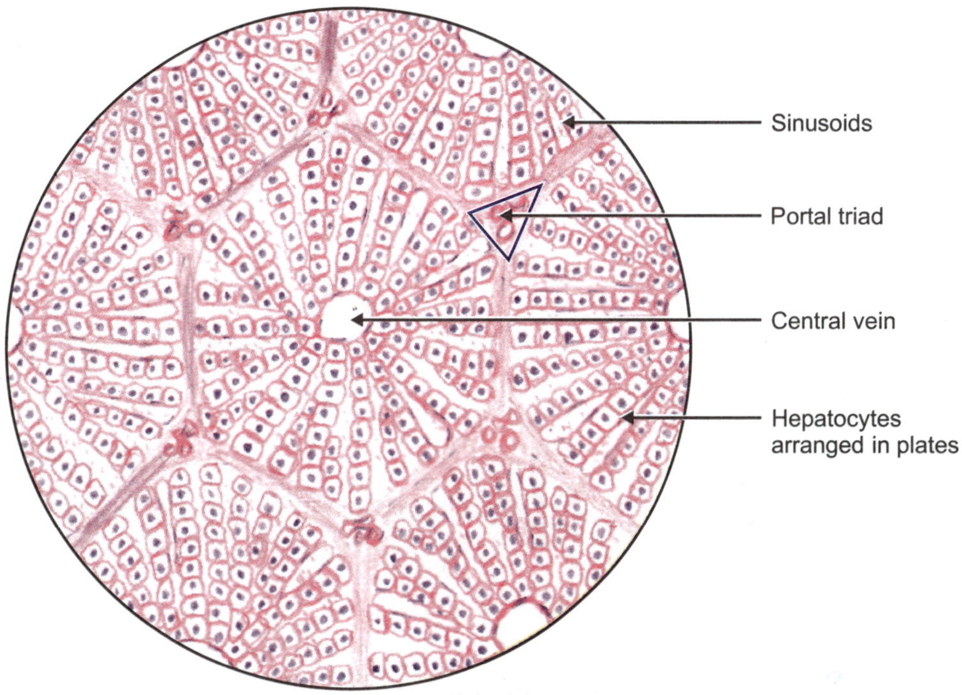
Sinusoids
Portal triad
Central vein
Hepatocytes
arranged in plates

GALLBLADDER

Mucosa: Lined by simple columnar epithelium with microvilli (brush border). Absence of goblet cells. Presence of lamina propria made up of connective tissue.

Muscularis mucosa and submucosa are absent.

Muscularis externa: It is a fibromuscular layer which consists of bundles of smooth muscle fibres oriented in different planes.

- In between the muscle fibres there is fibrous tissue rich in elastic fibres.

Serosa: Visceral peritoneum made up of a layer of loose connective tissue covered by mesothelium.

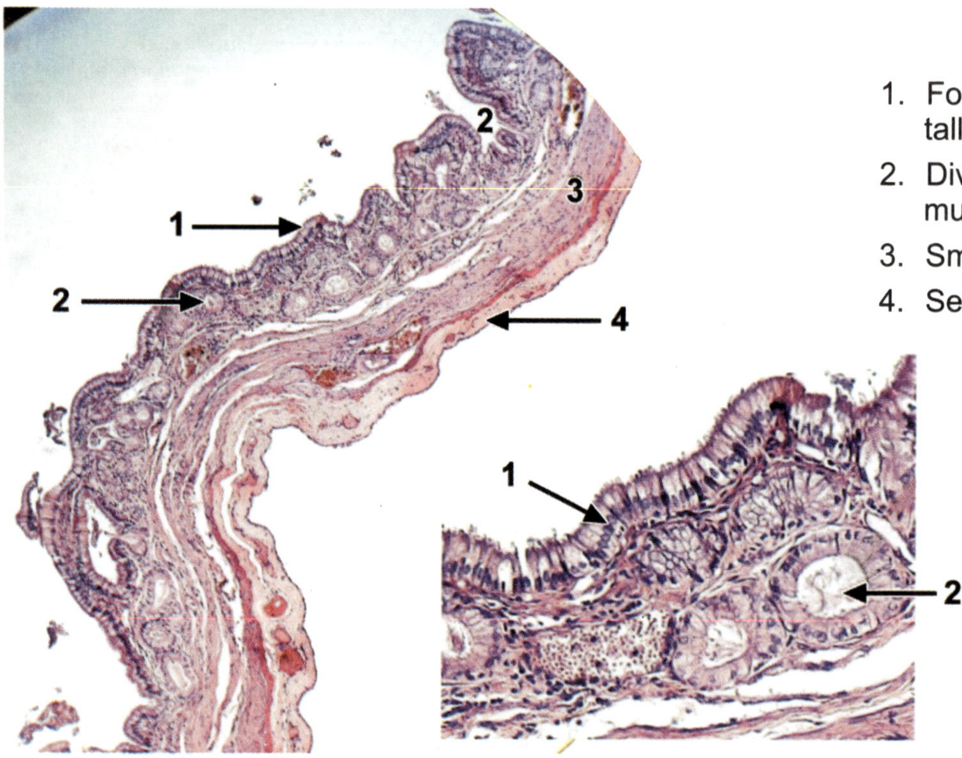

1. Fold in mucosa: Brush border tall columnar epithelium
2. Diverticulum or crypt of mucosa
3. Smooth muscle (muscularis)
4. Serosa

Key Features to Identify the Slide

- Mucosa lined by simple columnar epithelium with microvilli [brush border]
- Absence of submucosa and muscularis mucosa
- Fibromuscular coat is present

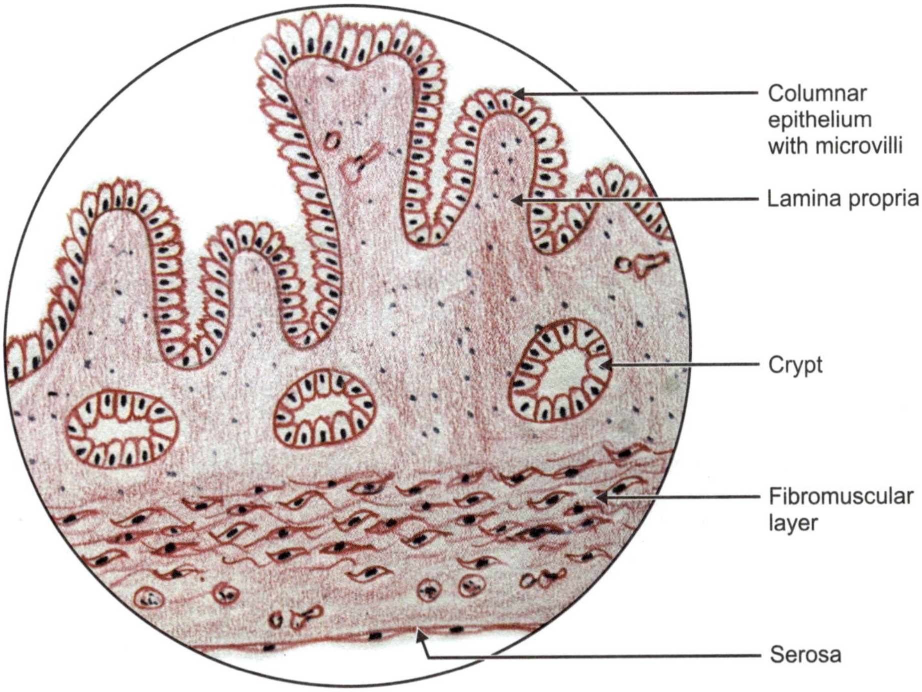
Columnar
epithelium
with microvilli
Lamina propria
Crypt
Fibromuscular
layer
Serosa

PANCREAS

Stroma: Pancreas is covered by connective tissue capsule from which septa arises and divide the gland into lobules.

Parenchyma: Pancreas being a mixed gland consists of both exocrine and endocrine parts.

Exocrine part: It is made up of pancreatic acini which are serous in nature. The cells of which resemble parotid gland exhibiting biphasic staining.

- Presence of extensive duct system. The one which begins within the lumen of the acinus is known as intercalated duct. They are lined by low cuboidal epithelium. These cells that lie within the acinus are called centroacinar cells.
- There are no striated ducts.
- Intercalated duct drains into intralobular duct lined by cuboidal epithelium.
- Intralobular duct drains into interlobular duct lined by simple columnar epithelium which lie in the connective tissue septa, they drain into main duct lined by tall columnar cells.

Endocrine part: Composed of small groups of cells called islets of Langerhans, they are scattered among the acini of the exocrine pancreas, they are lightly stained permeated by rich network of fenestrated capillaries.

The most numerous cells are alpha and beta, which secrete glucagon and insulin respectively.

- Less numerous cells are the delta cells which secrete somatostatin.
- F-cells secreting PP (pancreatic polypeptide).

Applied Aspects of Accessory Organs of Digestive System

1. Cirrhosis—it is progressive and irreversible damage of hepatocytes leading to fibrosis and most commonly due to alcoholic liver disease.
2. Acute pancreatitis—acute inflammation resulting in release of proenzymes causing necrosis of pancreatic cells due to infection, gallstones, alcoholism, drugs and trauma.

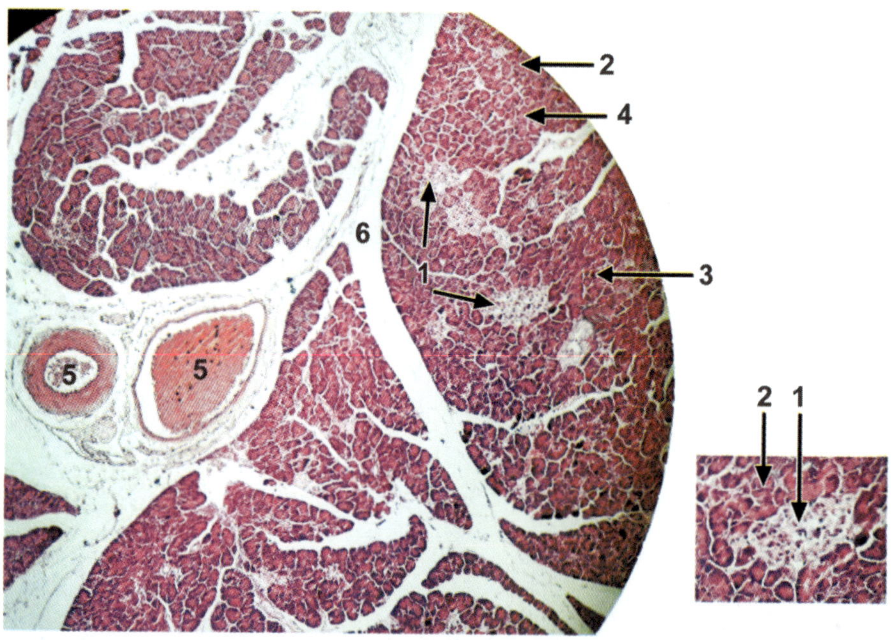

1. Islets of Langerhans (endocrine part)
2. Serous acini (exocrine part)
3. Intralobular duct
4. Centroacinar cell
5. Blood vessel
6. Interlobular connective tissue

Key Features to Identify the Slide

- Presence of numerous serous acini
- Lightly stained clusters of islets of Langerhans
- Presence of interlobular and intralobular ducts

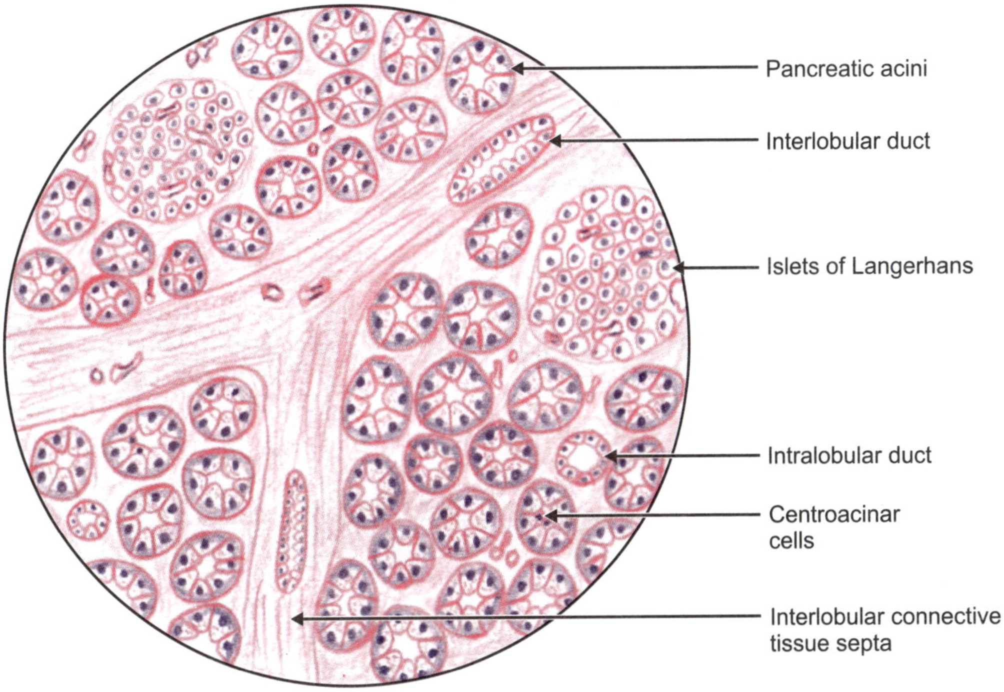
Pancreatic acini
Interlobular duct
Islets of Langerhans
Intralobular duct
Centroacinar cells
Interlobular connective tissue septa

QUESTIONS

1. Explain the structure of a hepatic lobule. 5M
2. What are Kupffer cells and their role. 2M
3. Describe the hepatic acinus. 5M
4. Discuss the features of the portal lobule in the liver. 5M
5. Elaborate on the significance of the space of Disse. 2M
6. What is space of Mall. 2M
7. Name the three components of the portal triad and highlight the one with the largest lumen. 2M
8. Explain the variations in acini found in salivary glands. 5M
9. Define and mention the functions of centroacinar cells. 2M
10. Outline the layers of the gallbladder wall. 2M
11. Name the different types of liver lobules. 2M
12. Microscopic anatomy of pancreas. 5M
13. Enumerate the different types of cells present in islets of Langerhans and mention their functions. 2M

Figures/Notes

KIDNEY (CORTEX)

Stroma: Consists of capsule and the connective tissue which support the nephrons and collecting system of ducts.

Parenchyma of cortex of kidney: Nephron being the structural and functional unit, is made up of:

(a) Renal corpuscles—which consists of Bowman's capsule and glomerulus.

(b) Proximal convoluted tubules—lined by simple cuboidal or low columnar epithelium with tall microvilli giving brush border appearance. The cytoplasm stains deeply with eosin.

(c) Loop of Henle: Lined by simple squamous epithelium and pale staining cytoplasm. It resembles a venule in cross section.

(d) Distal convoluted tubules—lined by cuboidal epithelium

- Absence of brush border and cytoplasm is stained lightly with eosin.

(e) Collecting tubules—they are wider in diameter, lined by cuboidal or low columnar epithelium.

Parenchyma of the medulla of the kidney: Shows sections of loop of Henle, collecting duct and plenty of capillaries.

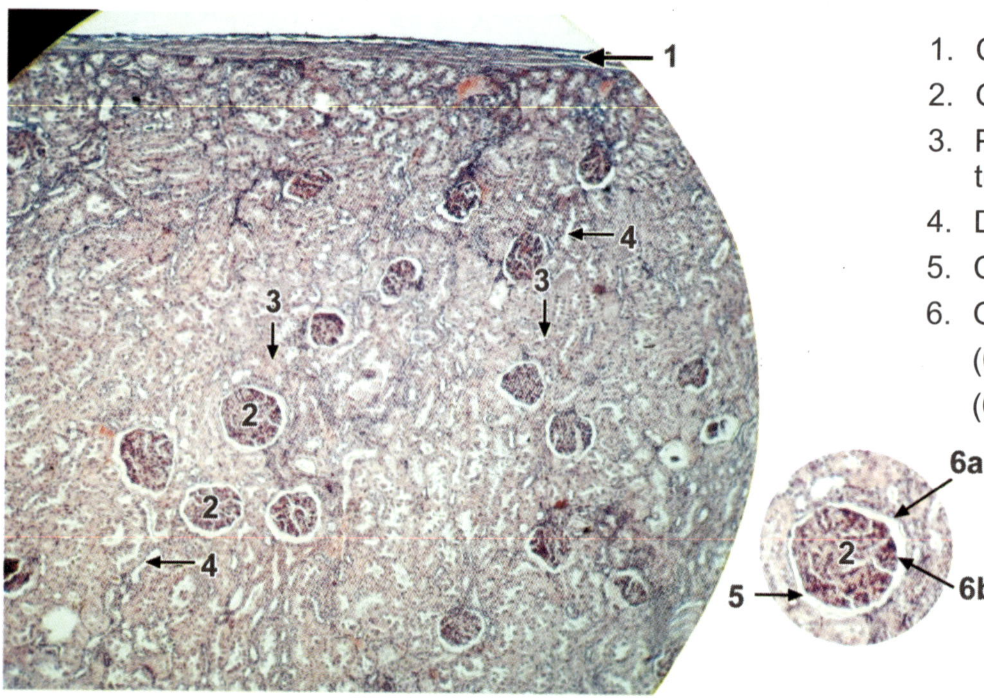

1. Capsule
2. Glomerulus
3. Proximal convoluted tubule
4. Distal convoluted tubule
5. Capsular space
6. Glomerular capsule
   (6a) Parietal layer
   (6b) Visceral layer

Key Features to Identify the Slide

- Presence of renal corpuscles, proximal and distal convoluted tubules in the cortex
- Presence of loop of Henle and collecting ducts in the medulla
- Presence of glomeruli surrounded by Bowman's capsule

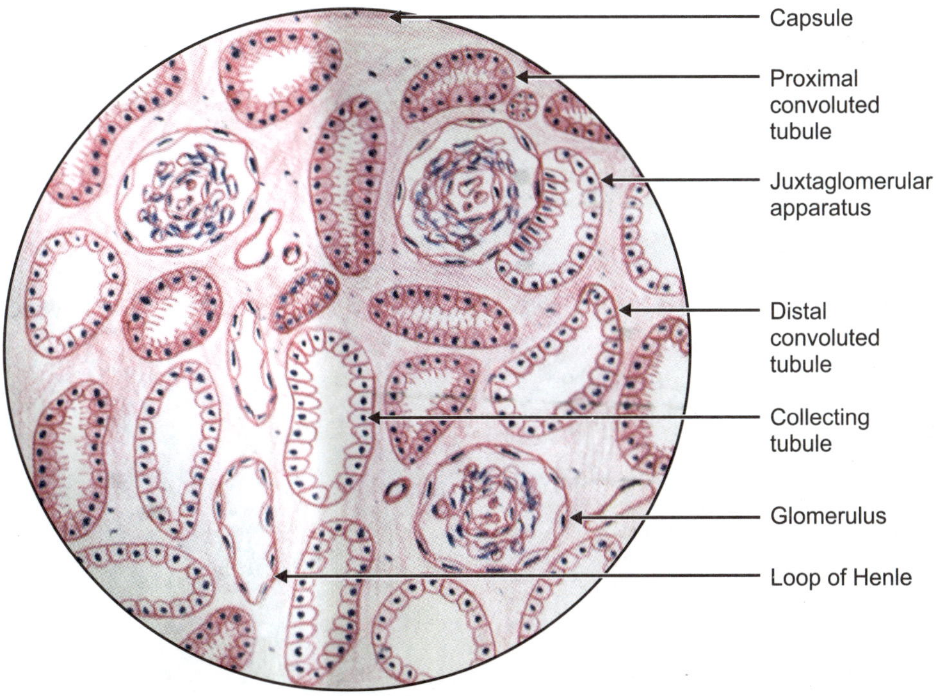
Capsule
Proximal convoluted tubule
Juxtaglomerular apparatus
Distal convoluted tubule
Collecting tubule
Glomerulus
Loop of Henle

URETER

Mucosa: Lined by transitional epithelium with underlying layer of lamina propria, made up of connective tissue.

Muscle layer: In upper part of inner longitudinal and outer circular layer.

- In middle and lower part, there is an additional outer longitudinal muscle layer.
- Adventitia—is made up of loose connective tissue containing many blood vessels.

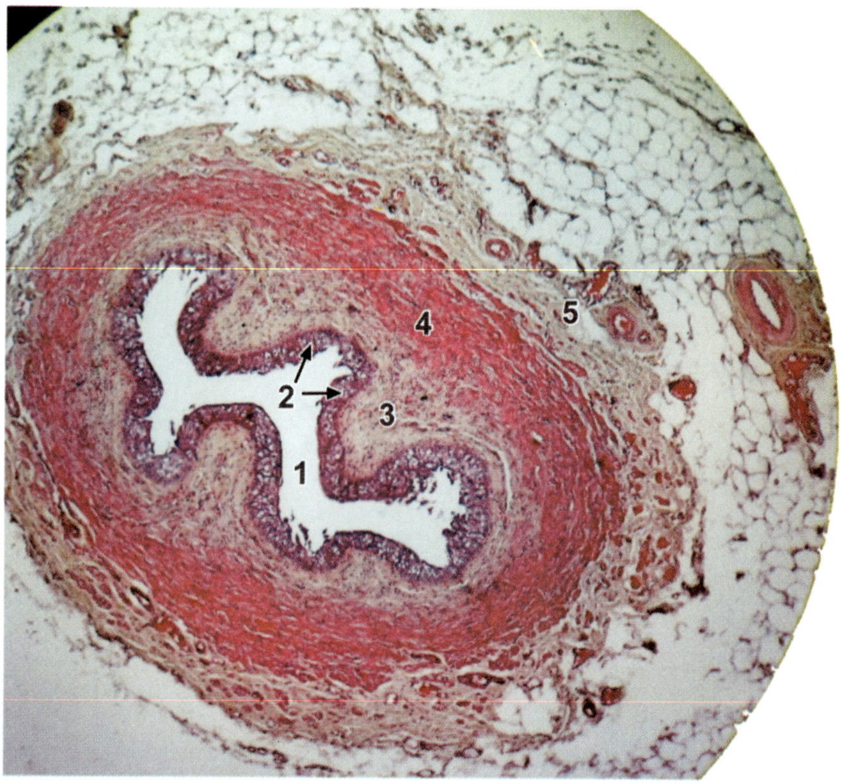

1. Lumen
2. Transitional epithelium
3. Lamina propria
4. Muscularis layer
5. Adventitia

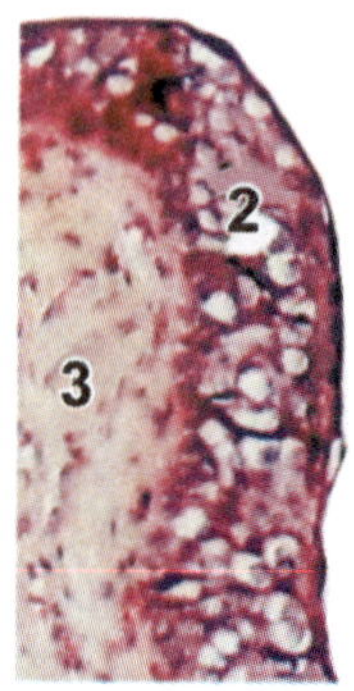

Key Features to Identify the Slide

- Mucous membrane is lined by transitional epithelium
- Lumen is star-shaped
- Presence of inner longitudinal and outer circular smooth muscle layers

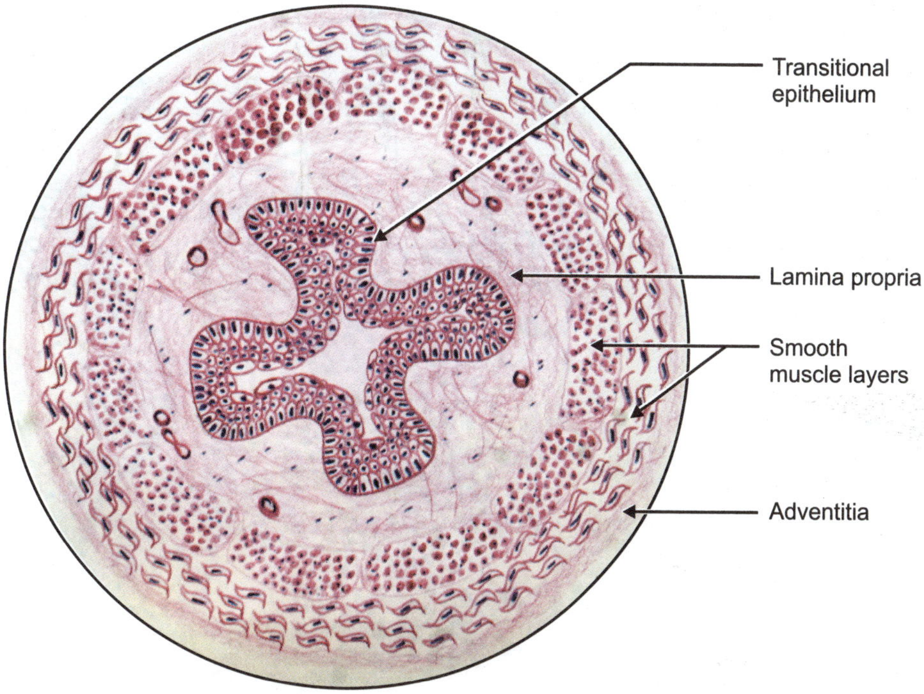
Transitional epithelium
Lamina propria
Smooth muscle layers
Adventitia

URINARY BLADDER

Mucosa: Lined by transitional epithelium (urothelium) with underlying lamina propria made up of connective tissue.

- The superficial cell layer takes up dark eosinophilic stain due to the presence of plaques (glycocalyx).

Muscle layer: Made up of thick smooth muscle coat with bundles of muscle fibres arranged in three indistinct layers, an inner and outer longitudinal and intermediate circular layer.

Serosa/Adventitia: The parts covered by peritoneum are lined by serosa; rest of the bladder being covered by adventitia made up of loose connective tissue.

Applied Aspects of Urinary System

1. Glomerulonephritis—inflammation of glomeruli leading to histological changes like thickening of basement membrane, leucocytic infiltration and deposition of immune complex.
2. Bladder carcinoma—arises from epithelial lining of urinary bladder and projects into the cavity of the bladder.

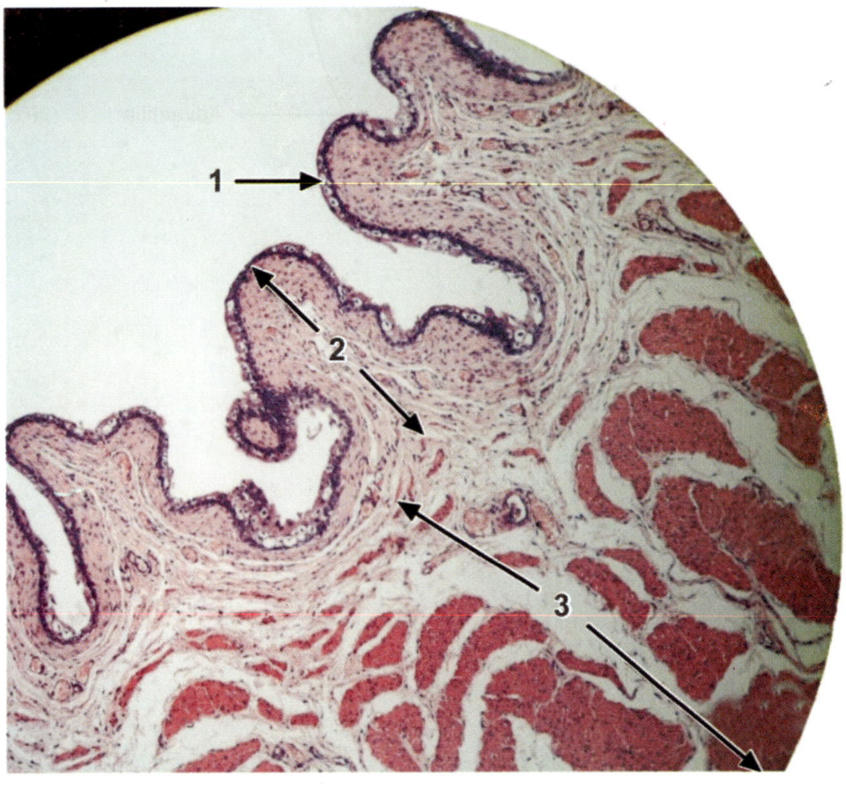

1. Transitional epithelium
2. Lamina propria
3. Smooth muscle bundles (sectioned in various planes)

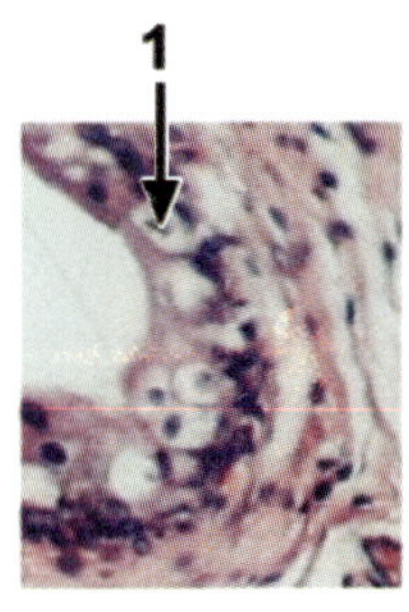

Key Features to Identify the Slide

- Mucous membrane lined by transitional epithelium
- Well-defined lamina propria beneath the mucosa
- Thick muscle coat running in different directions

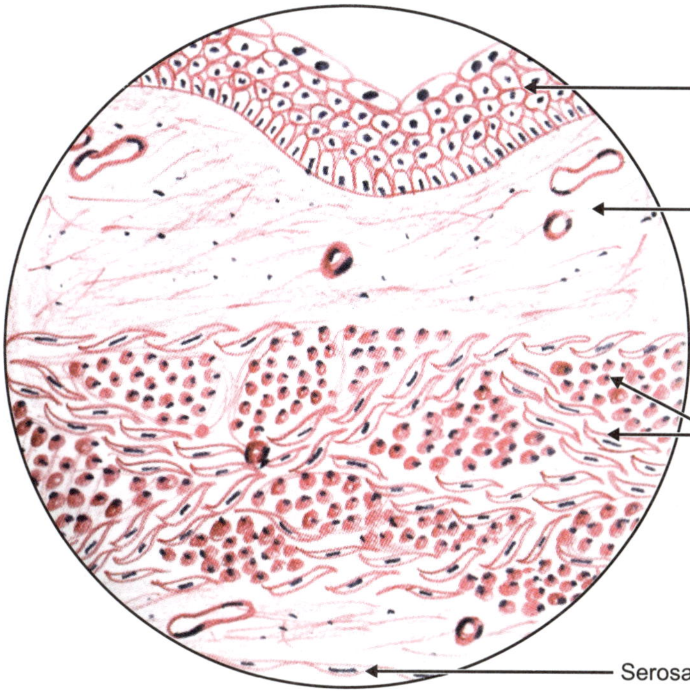
Transitional
epithelium
Lamina
propria
Smooth
muscle layers
Serosa

QUESTIONS

1. Explain in detail the components found in the cortex and medulla of a kidney. 5M
2. List the parts of a nephron and identify the cell types lining each section. 2M
3. Specify the lining epithelium of the ureter and urinary bladder. 2M
4. Differentiate between the two types of nephrons. 2M
5. Discuss the location, structure, and functional relationship of the juxtaglomerular apparatus. 5M
6. Microscopic differences between PCT and DCT. 5M
7. Explain the functions of urothelium. 2M

Figures/Notes

15 Male Reproductive System (AN 52.2)

TESTIS

Connective tissue capsule being contributed by tunica albuginea which is tough and collagenous in nature. It is posteriorly thickened to form mediastinum testis. Septa arises from the mediastinum and divide the parenchyma of the testis into approximately 250 lobules. Each lobule has 1–4 seminiferous tubules.

Seminiferous tubules: Sections of each seminiferous tubule surrounded by basal lamina on which a complex are stratified seminiferous epithelium rest. It is lined by two types of cells.

(a) Spermatogenic cells: They include spermatogonia (basally situated), spermatocytes, spermatids and mature spermatozoa involved in various stages of spermatogenesis.

(b) Sertoli cells: They are pyramid-shaped cells situated in between the spermatogenic cells, they provide mechanical and nutritive support to spermatogenic cells.

They are responsible for blood testis barrier .

The connective tissue between the seminiferous tubules contains Leydig cells in small clusters, they are polygonal and secrete testosterone. The connective tissue also contains fenestrated capillaries, nerves, lymphatics and peritubular myoid cells which are contractile in nature.

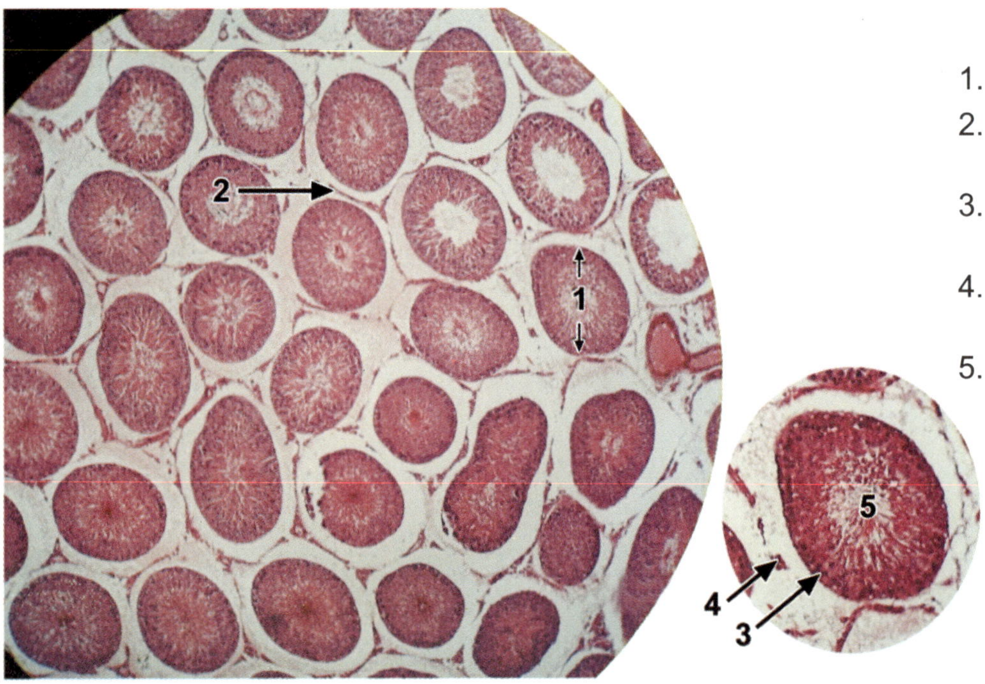

1. Seminiferous tubule
2. Interstitial connective tissue
3. Germinal epithelium with Sertoli cells
4. Interstitial cells of Leydig
5. Spermatid

Key Features to Identify the Slide

- Sections of numerous seminiferous tubules lined by cells of different stages of spermatocytes
- Presence of Sertoli cells
- Presence of interstitial cells of Leydig between the tubules

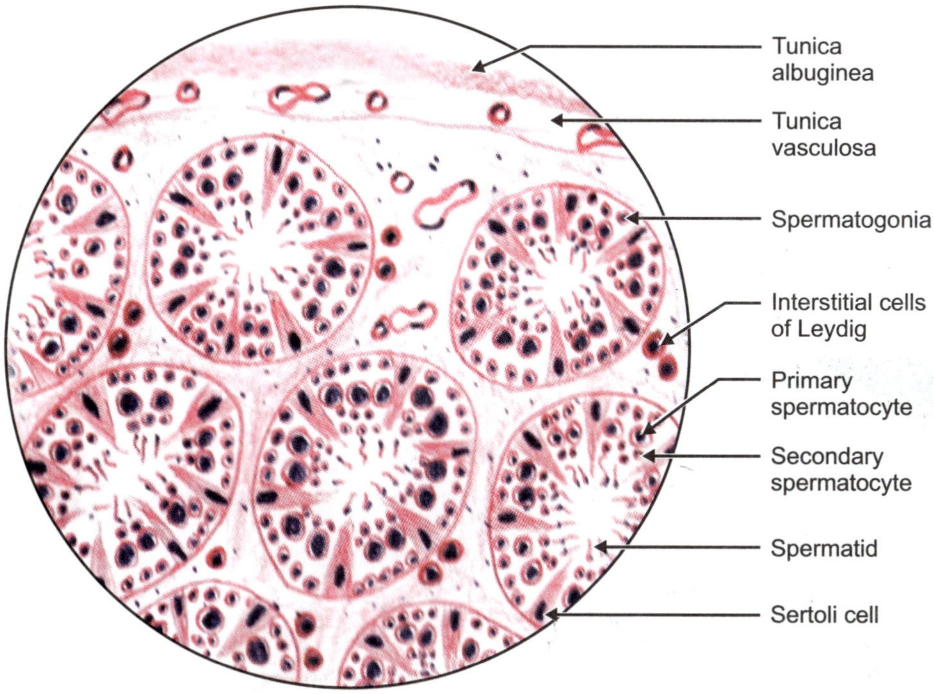
Tunica albuginea
Tunica vasculosa
Spermatogonia
Interstitial cells of Leydig
Primary spermatocyte
Secondary spermatocyte
Spermatid
Sertoli cell

EPIDIDYMIS

Epididymis is highly coiled tubular structure and the coils of tubules are surrounded by connective tissue.

The lining of tubules of epidermis is by pseudostratified columnar epithelium with stereocilia. In between the columnar cells and small basal cells are situated.

The lumen of the tubule may exhibit collected spermatozoa.

Beneath the basement membrane of the tubule a thin layer of circularly arranged smooth muscle fibres are noticed.

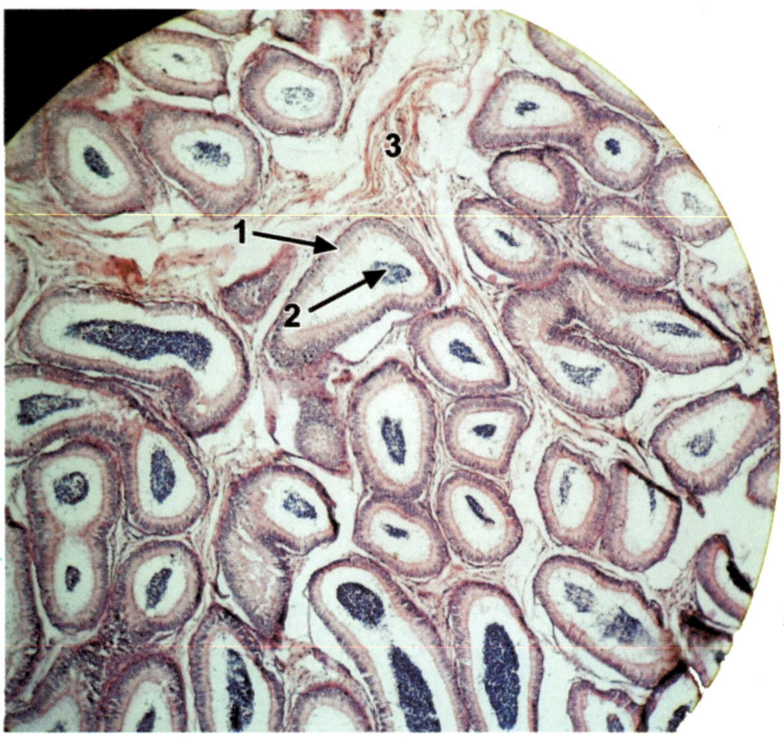

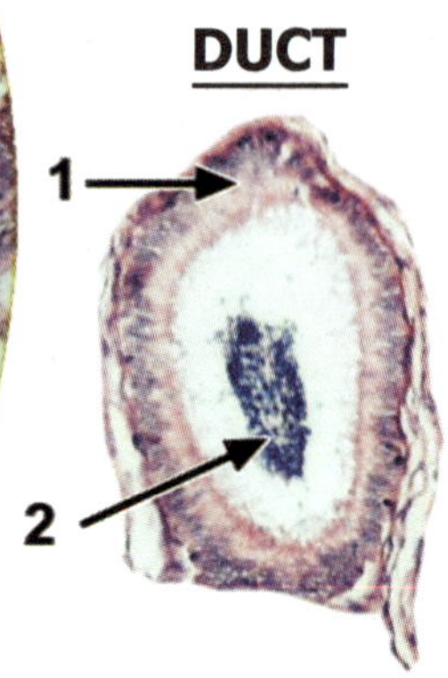

1. Pseudostratified epithelium with long nonmotile stereocilia
2. Clumps of sperms
3. Connective tissue

Key Features to Identify the Slide

- Duct lined by pseudostratified columnar epithelium with stereocilia
- Spermatozoa in lumen
- Smooth muscle layer surrounds each tubule

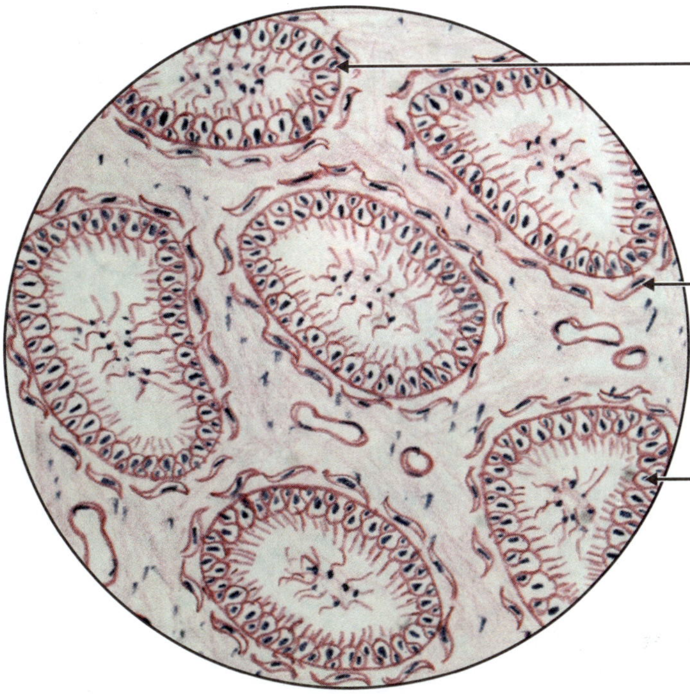
Tubule of epididymis
Smooth muscle layer
Pseudostratified columnar epithelium with stereocilia

DUCTUS (VAS) DEFERENS

Mucosa: Lined by pseudostratified columnar epithelium with stereocilia.

Muscle layer: It is thick and composed of smooth muscle fibres being arranged in inner longitudinal, middle circular and outer longitudinal layer.

Adventitia—made up of loose connective tissue containing blood vessels and nerves.

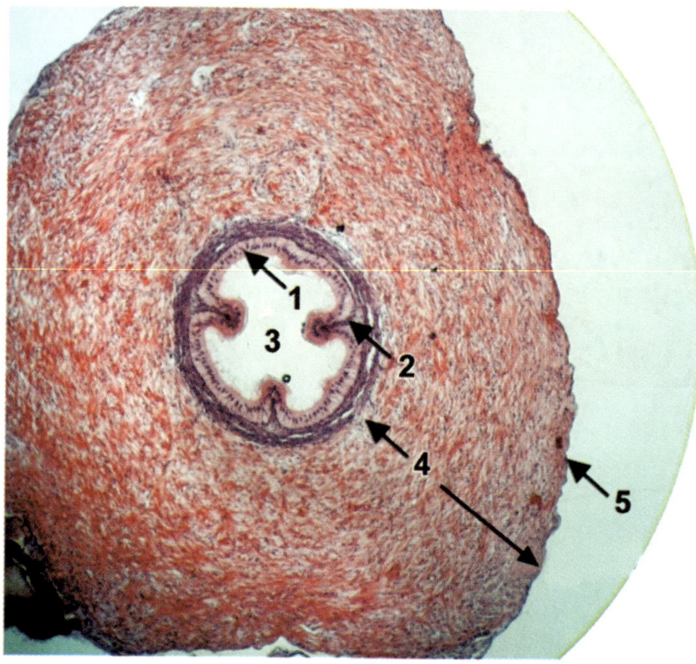

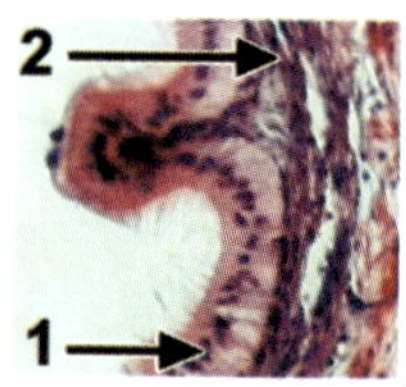

1. Pseudostratified columnar epithelium with stereocilia
2. Longitudinal crest of lamina propria
3. Narrow and irregular lumen
4. Thick muscularis (the inner longitudinal middle thick circular and thin outer longitudinal smooth muscle)
5. Adventitia

Key Features to Identify the Slide

- Presence of narrow lumen
- Lined by pseudostratified columnar epithelium with stereocilia
- Presence of thick inner longitudinal, middle circular and outer longitudinal muscle layers

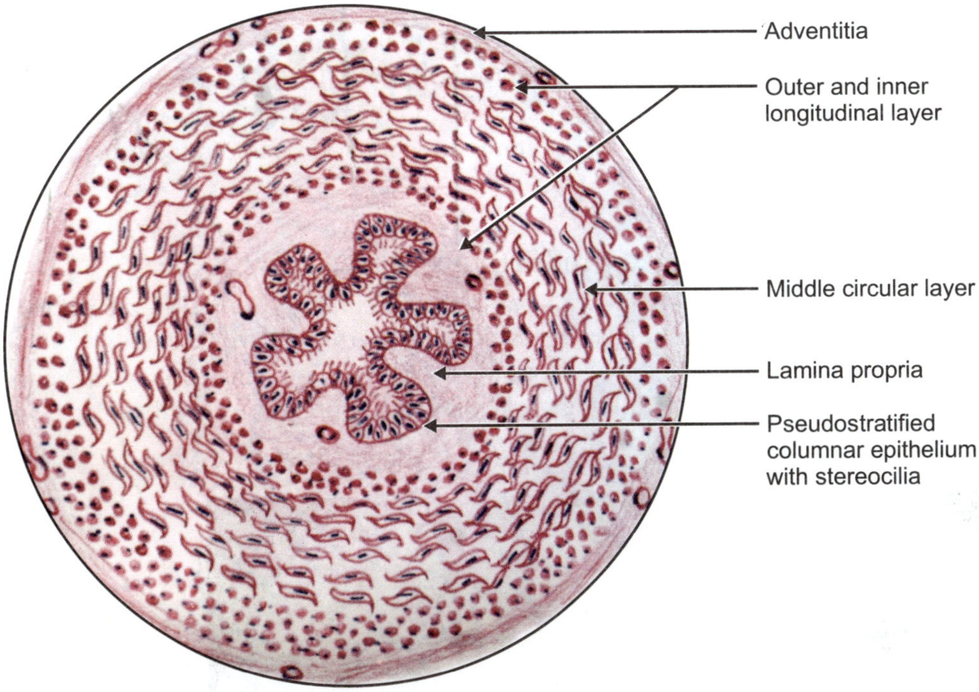
Adventitia
Outer and inner
longitudinal layer
Middle circular layer
Lamina propria
Pseudostratified
columnar epithelium
with stereocilia

PROSTATE

Stroma: The gland is covered by capsule and consists of fibromuscular tissue rich in collagen and elastic fibres with smooth muscle fibres in between them.

Parenchyma: Made up of tubuloalveolar gland, lined by simple cuboidal/columnar/pseudostratified columnar epithelium which varies depending on the activity of the gland.

The lumen of the acini may show an eosinophilic body called corpora amylacea or prostatic concretion, which are condensed secretory products seen in old people and they may become calcified.

The fibromuscular stroma run in different directions surrounding the acini and consists of blood vessels, lymphatics and nerves.

Applied Aspects of Male Reproductive System

1. Kartagener's syndrome—also termed as immotile cilia syndrome. The cilia of the spermatozoa and cells lining respiratory epithelium are defective resulting in infertility and bronchitis.
2. Benign prostatic hypertrophy—common condition affecting males above 50 years of age. There is enlargement due to proliferation of glandular tissue leading to compression of urethra.

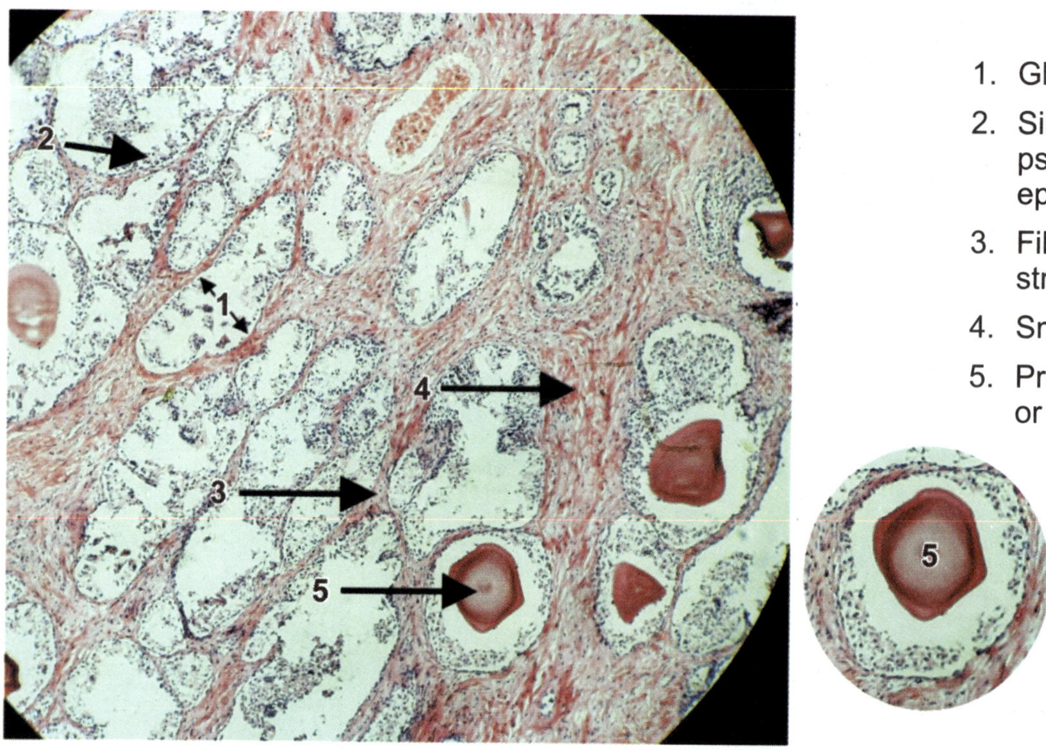

1. Glandular acini
2. Simple columnar or pseudostratified epithelium
3. Fibromuscular stroma
4. Smooth muscles
5. Prostatic concretion or corpora amylacea

Key Features to Identify the Slide

- Prostatic acini lined by simple columnar epithelium
- Presence of fibromuscular stroma
- Presence of corpora amylacea in the lumen

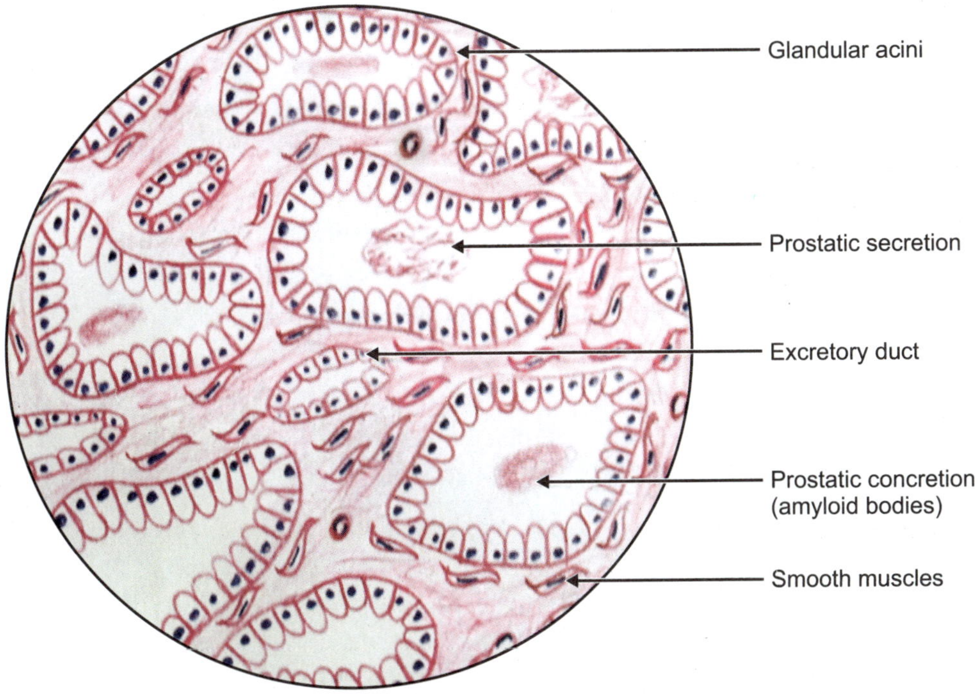
Glandular acini
Prostatic secretion
Excretory duct
Prostatic concretion
(amyloid bodies)
Smooth muscles

QUESTIONS

1. Explain the different stages of spermatogenesis. 5M
2. Microscopic structure of epididymis. 5M
3. Explain the concept of the blood-testis barrier. 5M
4. What is corpora amylacea? 2M
5. Where are the Sertoli cells located in the testis? Illustrate and list their functions. 5M
6. Define a testicular lobule and list its components. 2M
7. What are the stages of spermatogenesis? 2M
8. Outline the layers constituting the wall of vas deferens and their functions. 5M
9. What is the lining epithelium of the glands in the prostate? 2M
10. What are Leydig cells in the testis and mention their secretions. 2M

Figures/Notes

OVARY

Surface of the ovary: Covered by single layer of cuboidal epithelium called as germinal epithelium, but this is a misnomer because it is not the source of germ cells.

Beneath the epithelium the tunica albuginea is present which is a tough collagenous coat.

Cortex: Contains ovarian follicles of various stages of development along with corpora lutea and their degenerative remnants depending upon the age of the individual. These follicles are embedded in dense stroma composed of meshwork of collagen fibres and fusiform fibroblast like cells, arranged in characteristic whorls.

The stromal cells give rise to the thecal layers of maturing ovarian follicles.

Medulla: Highly vascular containing numerous veins and arteries within a loose connective tissue stroma

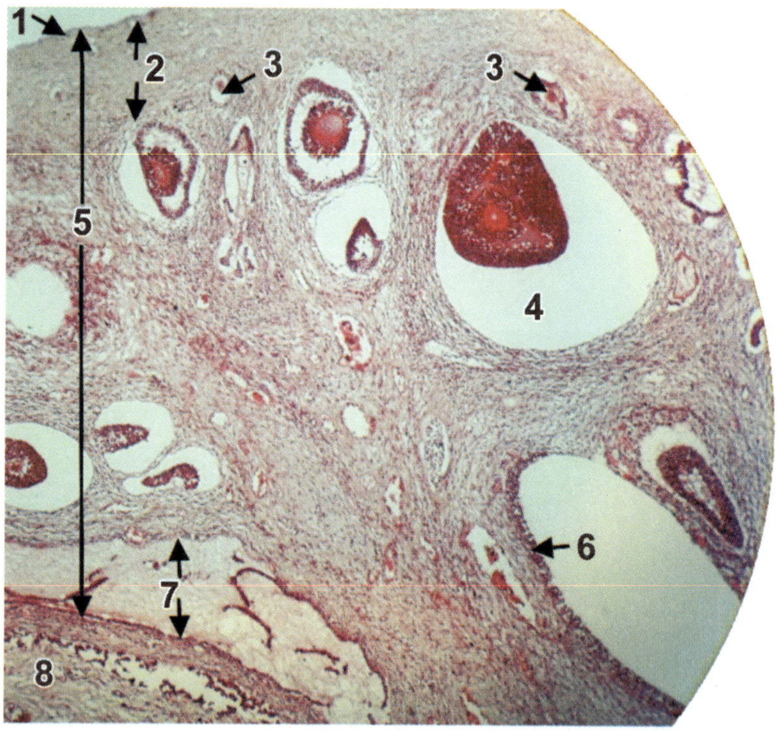

1. Germinal epithelium
2. Tunica albuginea
3. Primary follicle
4. Large mature follicle
5. Cortex
6. Vesicular (secondary) follicle: Granulosa cell
7. Atretic follicle
8. Medulla

Key Features to Identify the Slide

- Tunica albuginea with germinal epithelium
- Outer cortex shows different stages of ovarian follicles
- Presence of blood vessels and connective tissue in the medulla

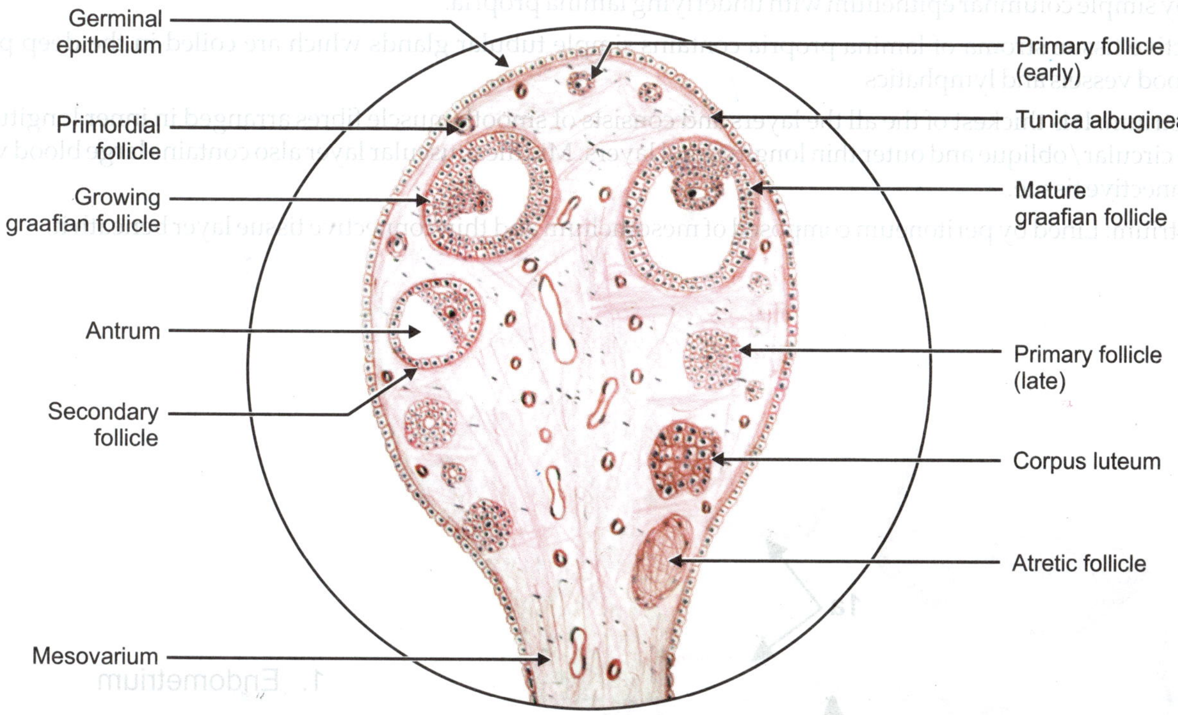
Germinal epithelium
Primordial follicle
Growing graafian follicle
Antrum
Secondary follicle
Mesovarium
Primary follicle (early)
Tunica albuginea
Mature graafian follicle
Primary follicle (late)
Corpus luteum
Atretic follicle

UTERUS: PROLIFERATIVE PHASE

Endometrium:

Lined by simple columnar epithelium with underlying lamina propria.

Connective tissue stroma of lamina propria contains simple tubular glands which are coiled in the deep portion with blood vessels and lymphatics

Myometrium: It is thickest of the all the layers and consists of smooth muscle fibres arranged in inner longitudinal, middle circular / oblique and outer thin longitudinal layers. Middle muscular layer also contains large blood vessels and connective tissue.

Perimetrium: Lined by peritoneum composed of mesothelium and thin connective tissue layer beneath it.

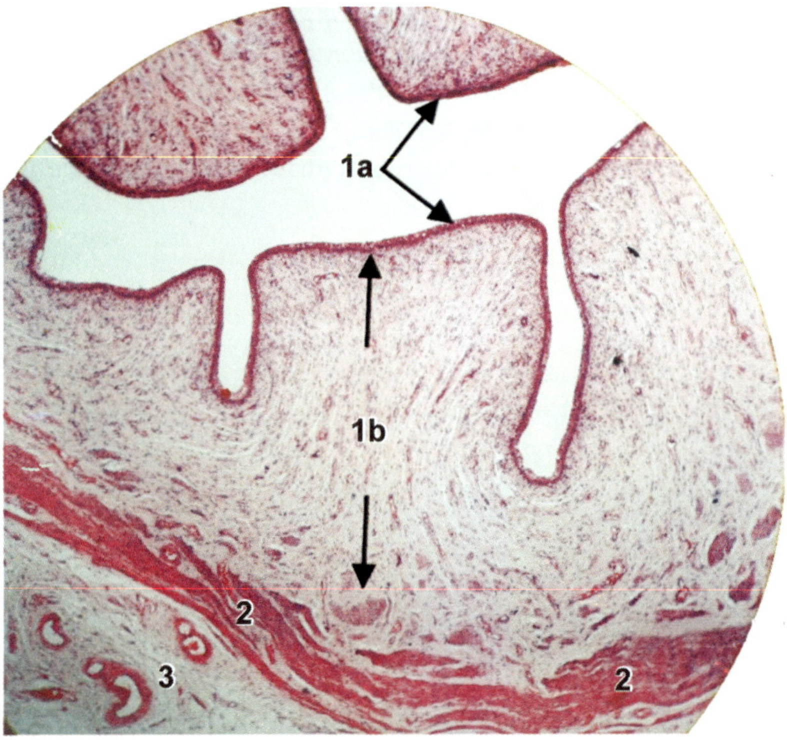

1. Endometrium
   1a. Simple columnar epithelium
   1b. Lamina propria
2. Myometrium
3. Perimetrium

Key Features to Identify the Slide

Uterus (proliferative phase)

- Endometrium lined by simple columnar epithelium
- Uterine glands in lamina propria
- Thick myometrium containing blood vessels

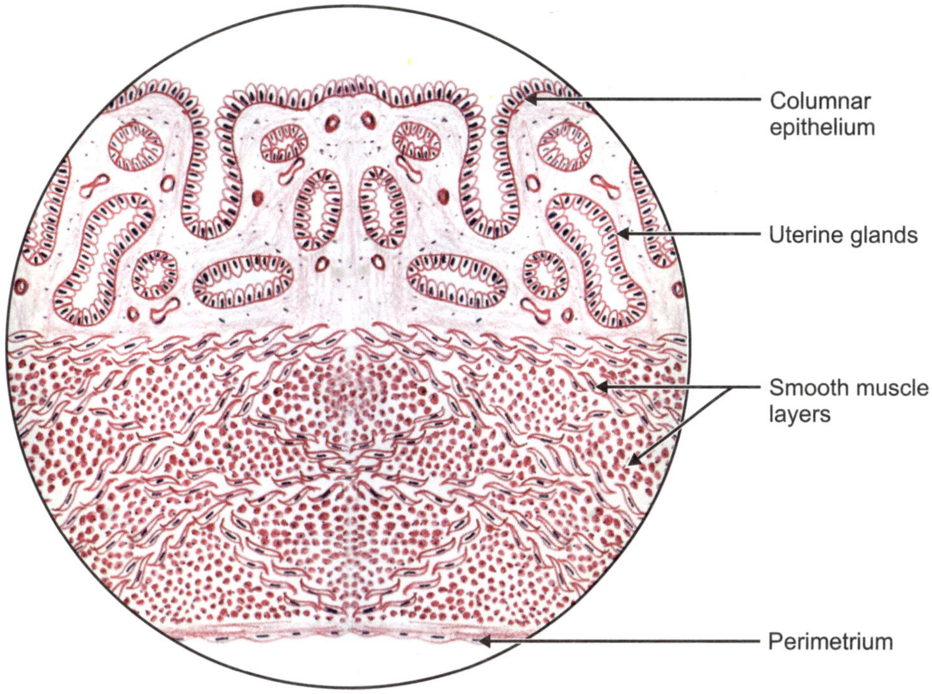
Columnar
epithelium
Uterine glands
Smooth muscle
layers
Perimetrium

UTERUS: SECRETORY PHASE

Endometrium:

Forms thick layer and contains endometrial glands which are tortuous due to increased accumulation of secretory products resulting in characteristic saw toothed appearance in sections. The spiral arteries are highly coiled and extend throughout the endometrium.

Myometrium: It is thickest of all the layers and consists of smooth muscle fibres arranged in inner longitudinal, middle circular/oblique and outer thin longitudinal layers. Middle muscular layer also contains large blood vessels and connective tissue.

Perimetrium: Lined by peritoneum composed of mesothelium and thin connective tissue layer beneath it.

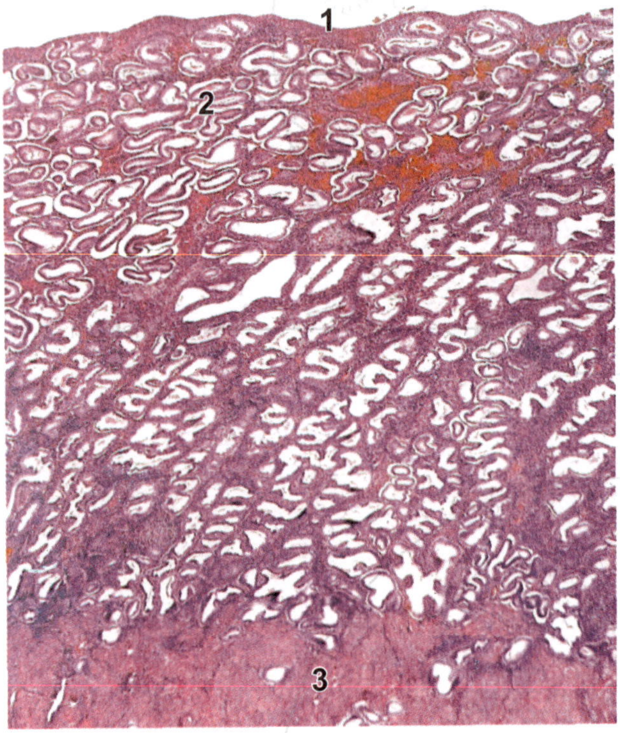

1. Columnar epithelium
2. Coiled uterine gland
3. Smooth muscle

Key Features to Identify the Slide

Uterus (secretory phase)

- Presence of thick layer of endometrium
- Tortuous glands in the lamina propria with characteristic saw-toothed appearance
- Spiral arteries seen extending throughout the length of endometrium

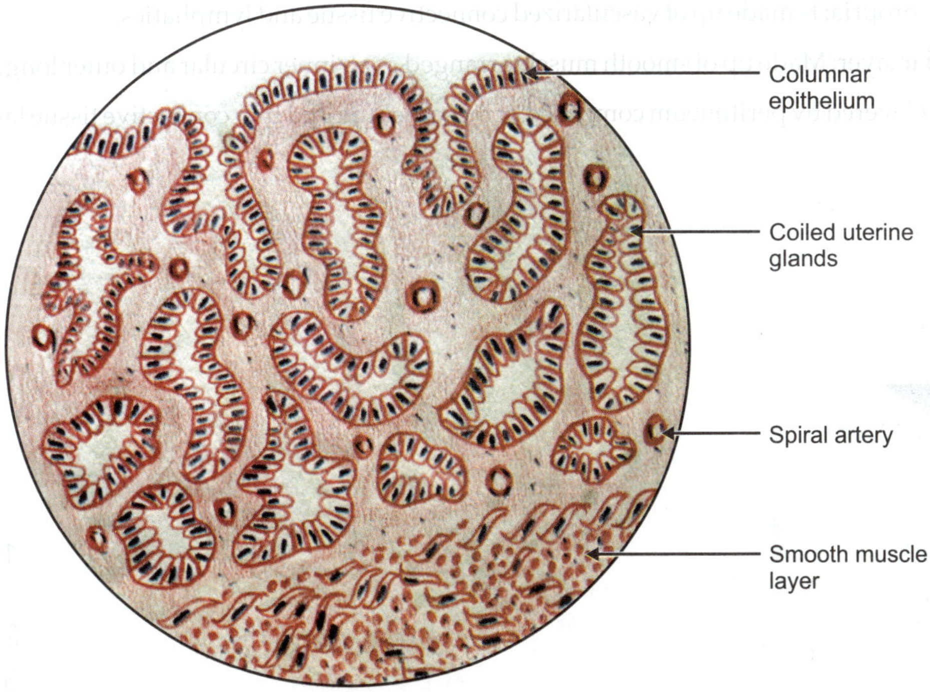
Columnar epithelium
Coiled uterine glands
Spiral artery
Smooth muscle layer

UTERINE TUBE/FALLOPIAN TUBE

Mucosa: Thrown into longitudinal folds lined by simple ciliated columnar epithelium with secretory cells in between them.

Lamina propria: Is made up of vascularized connective tissue and lymphatics.

Muscular layer: Made up of smooth muscle arranged as an inner circular and outer longitudinal layer.

Serosa: Covered by peritoneum composed of mesothelium and thin connective tissue layer beneath it.

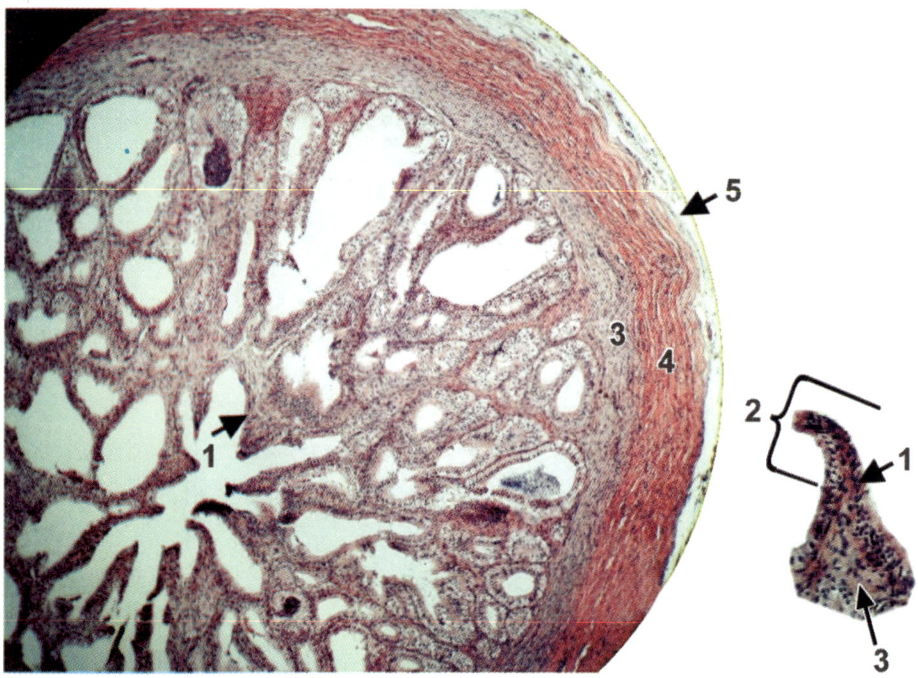

1. Ciliated columnar epithelium
2. Fold of mucosa
3. Lamina propria
4. Outer longitudinal and inner circular muscle fibres
5. Serosa (peritoneal mesothelium)

Key Features to Identify the Slide

- Mucous membrane thrown into folds
- Lined by simple ciliated columnar epithelium
- Inner circular and outer longitudinal muscle layers are seen

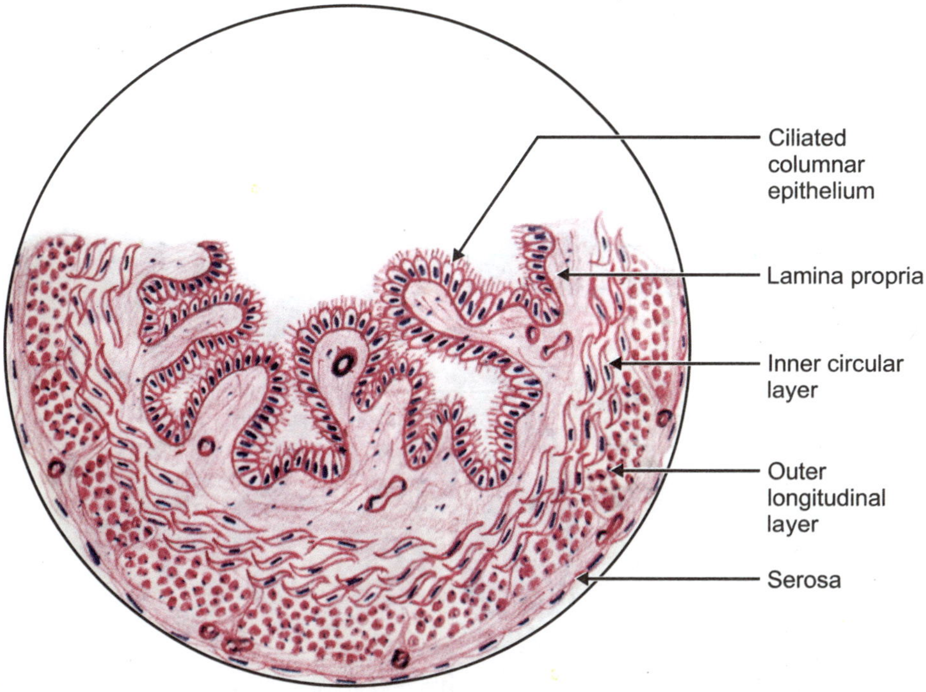
Ciliated columnar epithelium
Lamina propria
Inner circular layer
Outer longitudinal layer
Serosa

PLACENTA

Cross sections of chorionic villi exhibiting following features: Lined by inner layer of cytotrophoblast made up of cuboidal cells, lying on basement membrane.

Outer layer of syncytiotrophoblast made up of multinucleated cytoplasm with indistinct cell margins.

The core of the villi contains foetal capillaries within a layer of connective tissue derived from extraembryonic mesoderm. Presence of maternal blood along intervillous spaces. These layer forms placental barrier. The thickness of this barrier reduces during full term.

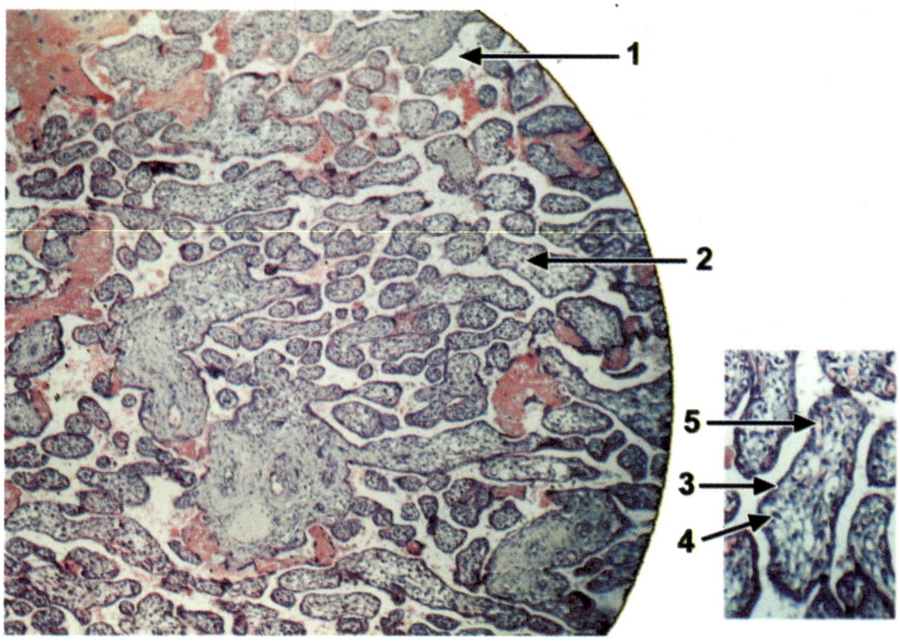

1. Intervillous space (maternal blood)
2. Villi with fetal blood vessels
3. Syncytiotrophoblasts
4. Cytotrophoblasts
5. Fetal blood vessels

Key Features to Identify the Slide

- Sections of chorionic villi are seen
- Villi are lined by syncytiotrophoblast and cytotrophoblast
- Foetal blood in capillaries
- Maternal blood in between the villi

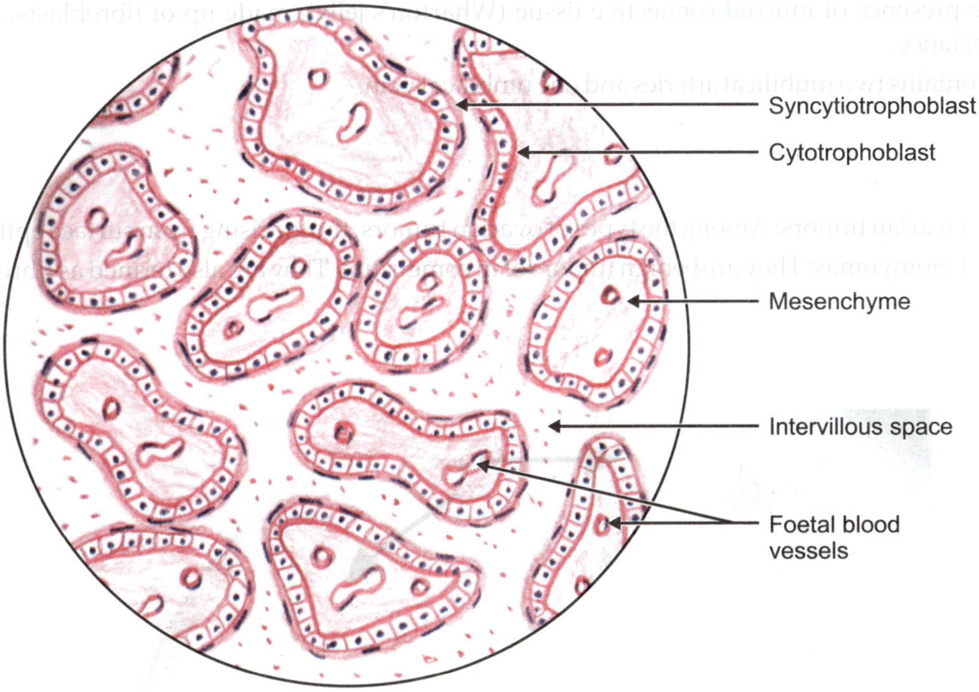
Syncytiotrophoblast
Cytotrophoblast
Mesenchyme
Intervillous space
Foetal blood vessels

UMBILICAL CORD

The cross section of umbilical cord shows: Amniotic membrane covering the umbilical cord lined by flattened epithelial cells.

The presence of mucoid connective tissue (Wharton's jelly), made up of fibroblasts, collagen fibres and ground substance.

It contains two umbilical arteries and one umbilical vein.

Applied Aspects of Female Reproductive System

1. Ovarian tumors: Among the types of ovarian tumors, those arising from surface epithelium are most common.
2. Leiomyomas: They are benign tumors of myometrium. They are also termed as fibroids.

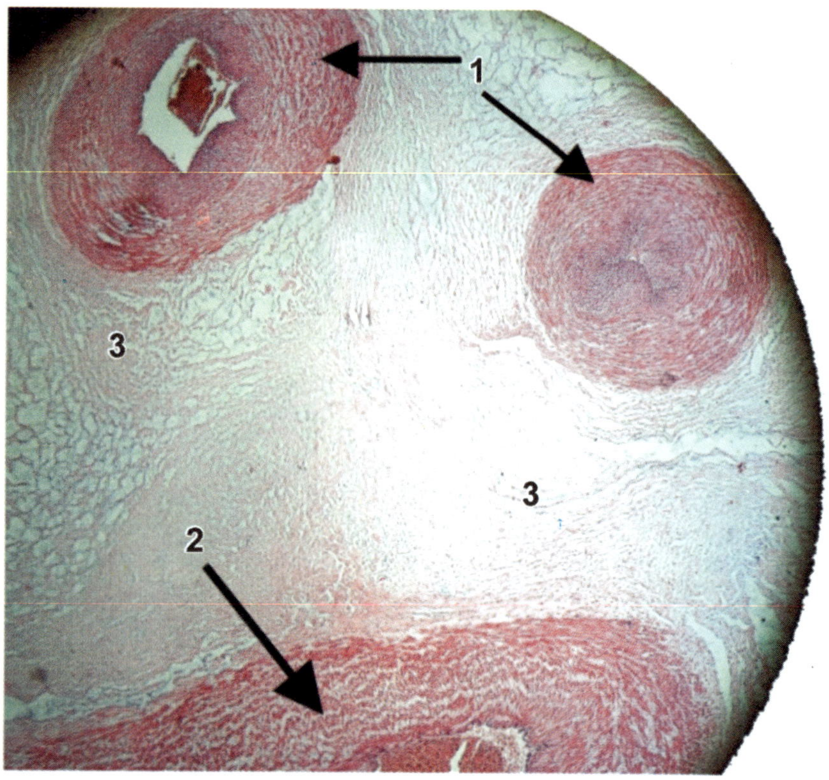

1. Umbilical arteries
2. Umbilical vein
3. Wharton's jelly

Key Features to Identify the Slide

- Presence of two umbilical arteries
- Presence of one umbilical vein
- Presence of Wharton's jelly

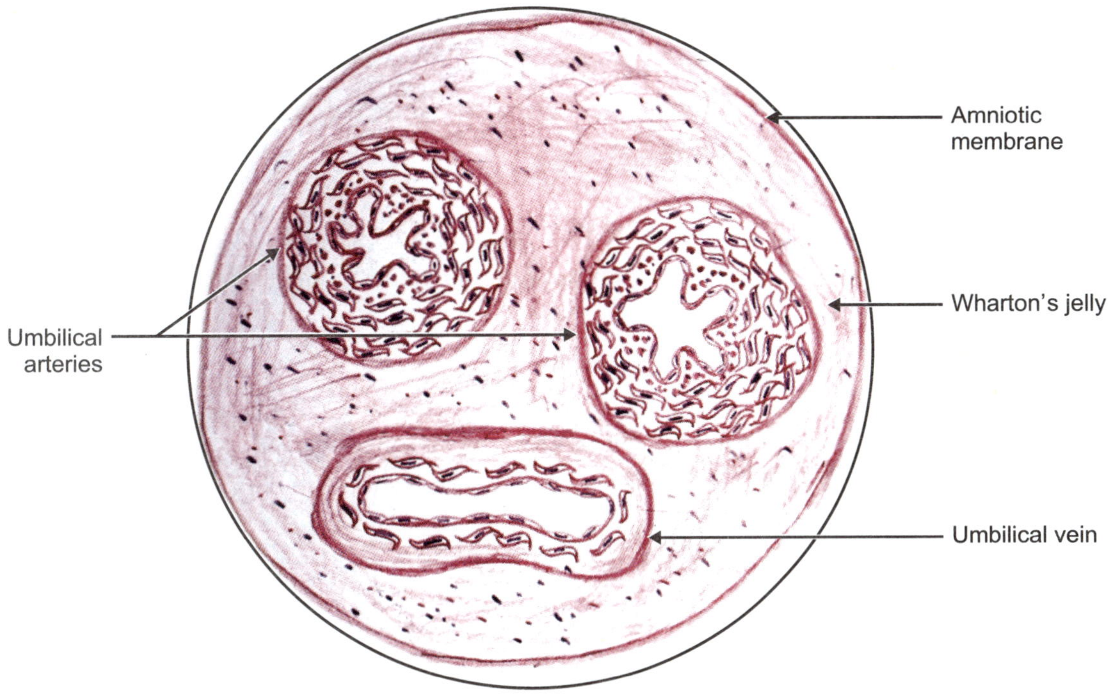
Amniotic membrane
Wharton's jelly
Umbilical arteries
Umbilical vein

QUESTIONS

1. What are the functions of corpus luteum. 2M
2. Compare the structure of various ovarian follicles. 5M
3. Identify different types of ducts in the mammary gland and their lining epithelium. 2M
4. Discuss the different layers of the wall of fallopian tube. 5M
5. Define uterine glands, their location, and changes during the menstrual cycle. 5M
6. List the layers constituting the uterine wall. 2M
7. What is zona pellucida? 2M
8. Explain about cumulus oophorus and corona radiata. 5M
9. Describe in detail microscopic changes in a lactating mammary gland compared to a resting one. 5M
10. Microscopic structure of mature ovarian follicle. 5M
11. Discuss the microscopic features of the umbilical cord. 5M
12. Mention the functions of Wharton's jelly. 2M
13. Explain the microscopic structure of the placenta and outline its functions. 5M
14. Define the placental barrier and discuss its clinical significance. 5M

Figures/Notes

PITUITARY GLAND

Adenohypophysis/Pars anterior/Distalis: Consists of two types of secretory cells arranged in clumps or irregular cords between the network of capillaries. They are supported by network of connective tissue.

(a) Chromophils—classified as acidophils which stain pink (eosinophilic) and basophils which stain blue (basophilic).

- Acidophils secrete growth hormone and prolactin. Basophils secrete TSH, FSH, LH and ACTH.

(b) Chromophobes—they are poorly stained as they contain very few secretory granules.

Pars intermedia: Presence of cysts containing colloid lined by cuboidal cells. It contains basophilic cells which secrete MSH.

Neurohypophysis/Pars posterior: Consists of unmyelinated axons of neurons located in supraoptic and paraventricular nuclei. It also contains pituicytes which are supporting neuroglial cells.

Presence of Herring bodies which are collection of secretory granules at the terminal portion of axonal processes. They contain two hormones: Oxytocin and vasopressin (ADH) that are released into the capillaries.

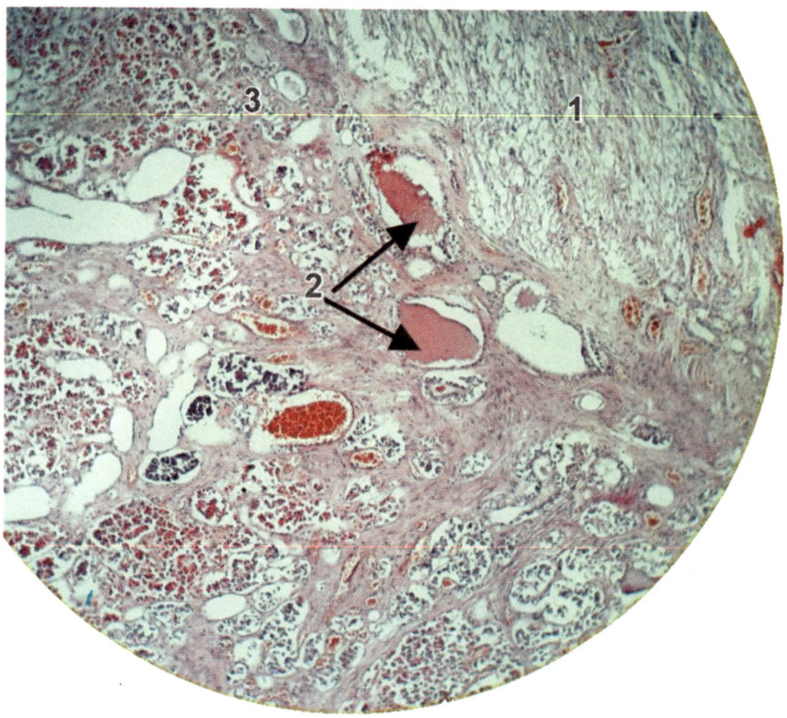

1. Pars nervosa
2. Pars intermedia with colloid vesicles
3. Pars anterior

Key Features to Identify the Slide

- Presence of chromophils and chromophobes in pars anterior
- Presence of pituicytes and nerve fibres in pars posterior
- Presence of colloidal vesicles in pars intermedia

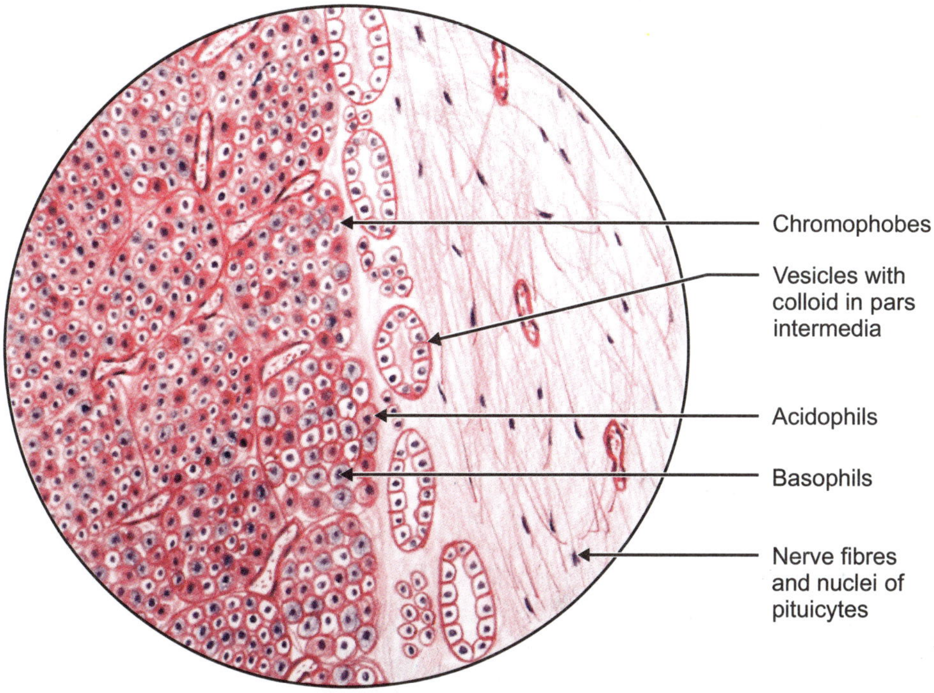
Chromophobes
Vesicles with colloid in pars intermedia
Acidophils
Basophils
Nerve fibres and nuclei of pituicytes

THYROID AND PARATHYROID GLANDS

Thyroid

Stroma: Covered by connective tissue capsule, which sends septa into the gland dividing each lobe into irregular-shaped lobules. The septa also convey the blood vessels, nerves and lymphatics into the gland.

Parenchyma: Consists of follicles which are the functional unit of thyroid gland. Wall of the follicle is lined by simple cuboidal epithelium but the shape of the cells varies depending upon the functional activity of the gland. Follicles are surrounded by delicate connective tissue stroma containing fenestrated capillaries. The lumen of the follicle is filled with colloid (iodinated thyroglobulin), which takes up eosinophilic stain.

Presence of parafollicular or C-cells embedded within the follicles or in between the follicles in the form of clusters in the interfollicular stroma. These cells secrete calcitonin.

Parathyroid

Covered by thin connective tissue capsule. Consists of two main types of cells.

(a) Chief cells/principal cells—most numerous polygonal-shaped cells which are small-sized arranged in clumps or irregular cords.

Presence of capillaries in between the cords of the cells. They secrete parathormone.

(b) Oxyphil cells—they are less numerous than chief cells but are larger in size. Cytoplasm stains deeply with eosin. They are arranged in small clumps. Their functional significance is uncertain.

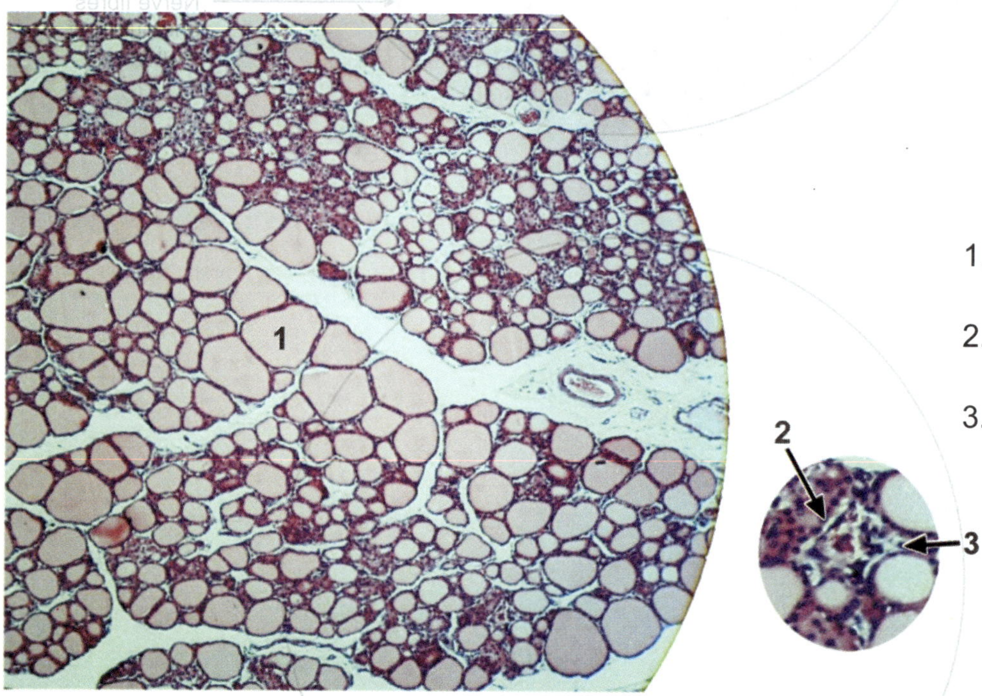

1. Follicles with colloid
2. Simple cuboidal epithelium
3. Parafollicular cell

Key Features to Identify the Slide

- Presence of thyroid follicles lined by cuboidal cells
- Follicles are filled with colloid
- Presence of parathyroid gland showing chief and oxyphil cells

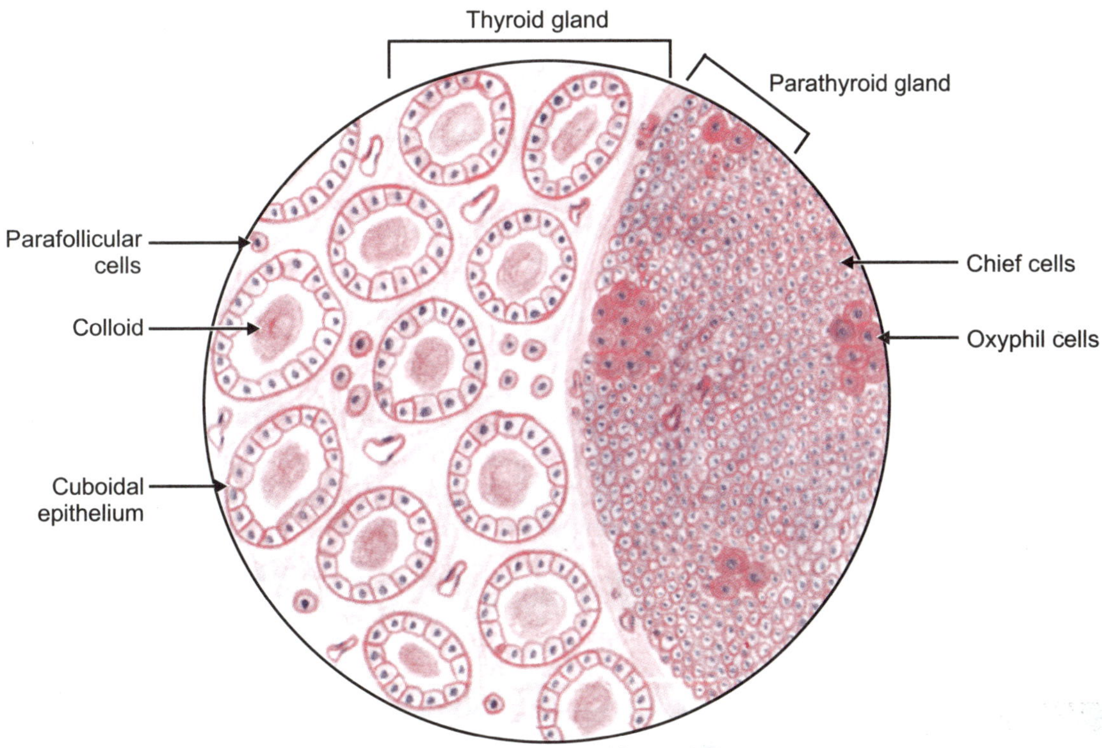
Thyroid gland
Parathyroid gland
Parafollicular cells
Colloid
Cuboidal epithelium
Chief cells
Oxyphil cells

ADRENAL/SUPRARENAL GLAND

Stroma: Covered by connective tissue capsule which sends septa towards the interior of the gland carrying vessels and nerves.

Parenchyma:

Adrenal cortex—consists of three zones:

(a) Zona glomerulosa—made up of small polyhedral cells in rounded clusters. The cells have basophilic cytoplasm containing a few lipid droplets and deep staining nucleus.

They secrete—aldosterone.

(b) Zona fasciculata—this broader intermediate layer consists of large polyhedral basophilic cells, arranged in straight columns two cells wide with parallel fenestrated capillaries in between them. The cells contain many lipid droplets, so the cytoplasm appears vacuolated. Hence, these cells are called spongiocytes.

They secrete—glucocorticoids (cortisol).

(c) Zona reticularis—consists of branching interconnected columns of rounded cells whose cytoplasm contains aggregates of brown lipofuscin pigment that accumulate with age.

They secrete—androgens.

Adrenal medulla: Composed of groups and columns of chromaffin cells (pheochromocytes) separated by capillaries and supported by a network of reticular fibres. Functionally they are equivalent to postganglionic sympathetic neurons and release adrenaline and noradrenaline.

Applied Aspects of Endocrine System

1. Pituitary adenoma: It is most common benign tumor of pituitary gland resulting in excessive secretion of hormones.
2. Goitre: It is enlargement of thyroid gland due to various causes like tumor, inflammation and iodine deficiency.

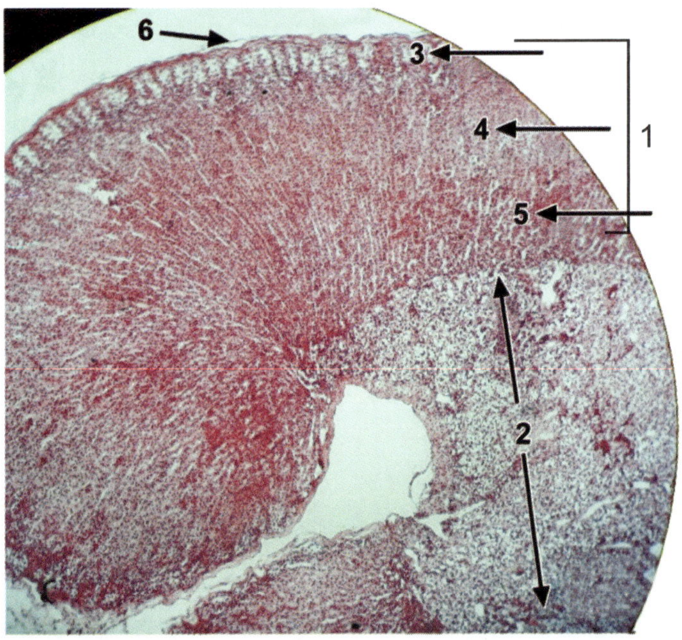

1. Cortex
2. Medulla (chromaffin)
3. Zona glomerulosa
4. Zona fasciculata
5. Zona reticularis
6. Capsule

Key Features to Identify the Slide

- Capsule with trabeculae
- Cortex showing zona glomerulosa, zona fasciculata and zona reticularis
- Presence of chromaffin cells and sinusoids in medulla

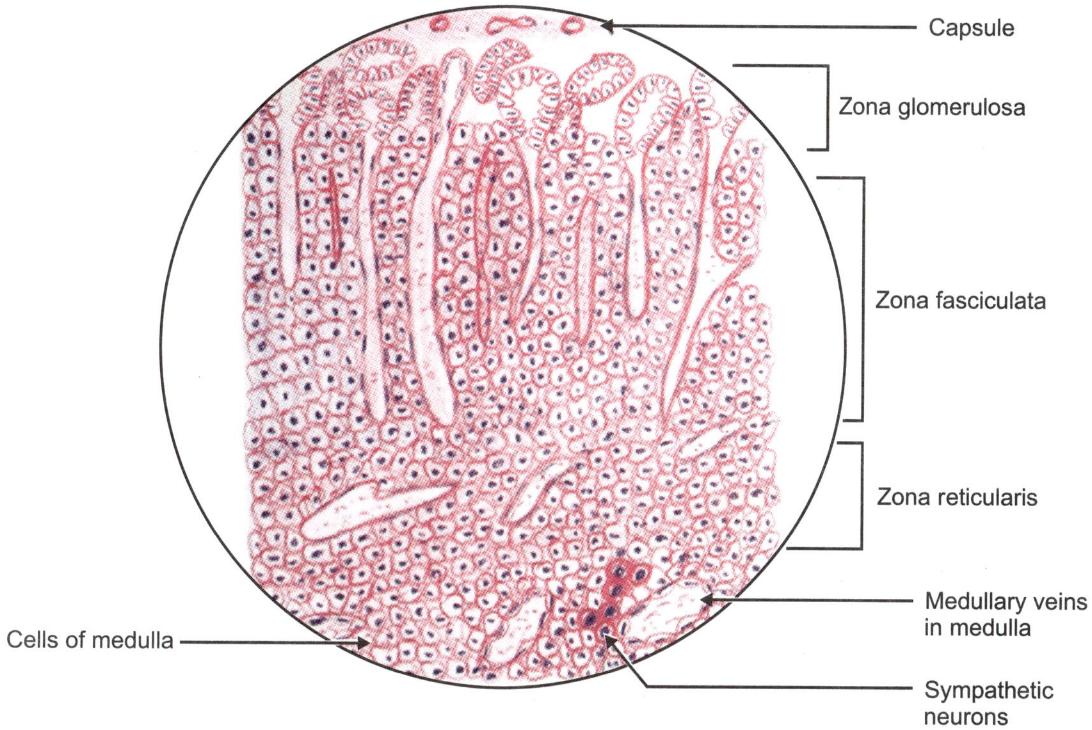
Capsule
Zona glomerulosa
Zona fasciculata
Zona reticularis
Medullary veins in medulla
Cells of medulla
Sympathetic neurons

QUESTIONS

1. List the types and features of cells present in the anterior pituitary gland and elaborate on their functions. 5M
2. Describe the histology of adrenal gland. 5M
3. Microanatomy of pituitary gland. 5M
4. Explain the features of thyroid follicles and distinguish between active and inactive ones. 5M
5. Define the features of cells in the parathyroid gland and discuss their functions. 5M
6. Describe the microscopic structure and function of a thyroid follicle. 5M
7. What are Herring bodies? 2M
8. Define the characteristic features of the pars intermedia in the pituitary gland. 2M
9. What are parafollicular cells and their functions. 2M
10. What is chromaffin reaction? 2M

Figures/Notes

CEREBRUM

Cerebral cortex exhibits 6 layers with no proper distinction between the layers. They are arranged in following layers from superficial to deep:

1. Molecular layer/plexiform layer—situated beneath the pia mater consists predominantly of fibres and neuroglial cells. Presence of few horizontal cell of Cajal.
2. External granular layer—consists of varying density of small neuronal cell bodies of pyramidal cells and granular (stellate) cells. However, the granular cells are predominant.
3. External pyramidal layer—consists of medium-sized pyramidal cells with their processes. Other cells present in this layer are cells of Martinotti and stellate cells.
4. Internal granular layer—narrowest of all the layers, consists of densely packed granular cells with some pyramidal cells.

Presence of a prominent band of horizontal fibres called external band of Baillarger.

5. Internal pyramidal layer—consists typically of largest pyramidal cells (of Betz). This layer is traversed by a prominent central band of horizontal fibres (inner band of Baillarger).
6. Multiform/fusiform (pleiomorphic) layer—consists of neurons with a variety of shapes. The spindle-shaped fusiform cells are predominant.

Deep to this layer of cerebral cortex lies the white matter.

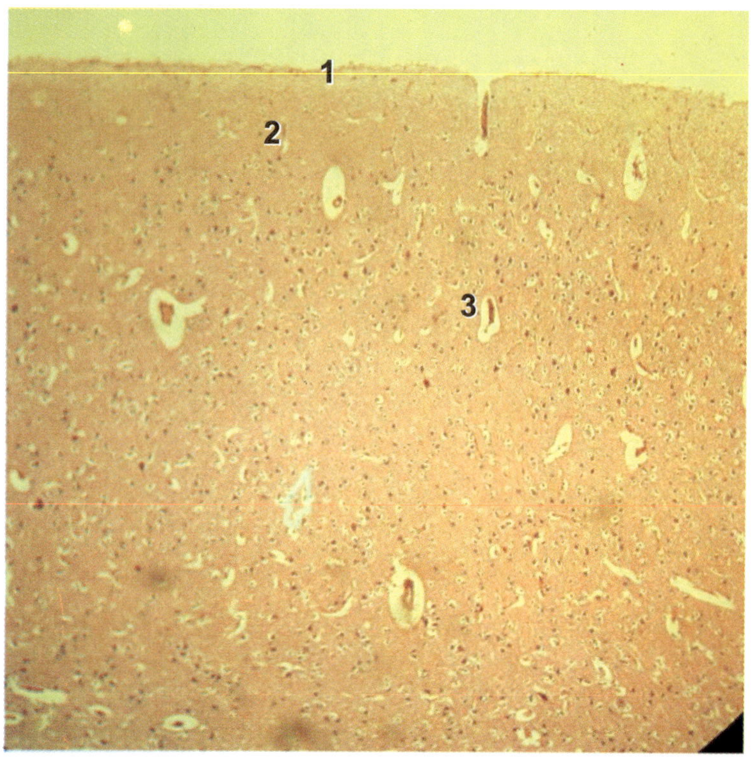

1. Pia mater
2. Granule cell
3. Pyramidal cell

Key Features to Identify the Slide

- Pyramidal and stellate cells are present
- Outer layer is pia mater
- Myelinated nerve fibres in medulla

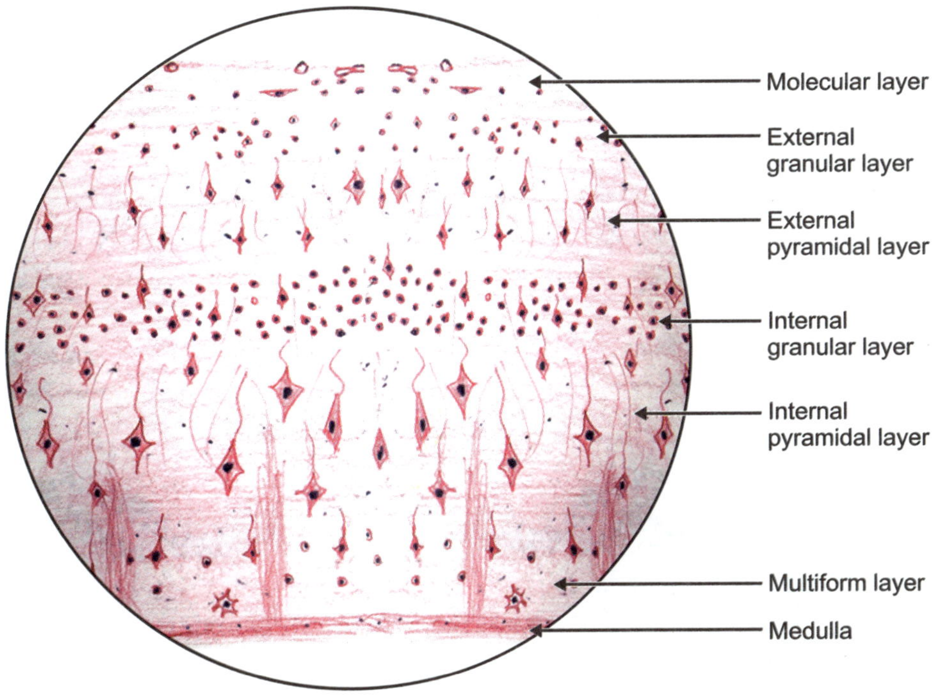
Molecular layer
External granular layer
External pyramidal layer
Internal granular layer
Internal pyramidal layer
Multiform layer
Medulla

CEREBELLUM

The cerebellar cortex consists of three layers that are as follows from superficial to deep:

1. Molecular layer—it is situated beneath the pia mater consists of few cells and more number of fibres. The cells found in this layer are—basket cells and stellate cells.

Most of the layer is occupied by dendritic processes of Purkinje and Golgi cells and external processes of granular cells. It also contains terminal part of climbing fibres.

2. Purkinje cell layer—contains large pear-shaped (flask-shaped) cell bodies of Purkinje cells. Each cell gives rise to fan-like dendritic tree which extends into the molecular layer. The axon of these cells arises from its base and pass through the granular layer to enter the white matter.
3. Granular layer—consists of somata of densely packed granular cells. They form synaptic contact with mossy fibres.

This layer also contains Golgi cells, the dendrites of which extend into the molecular layer.

Deep to this layer of cerebellar cortex lies the white matter.

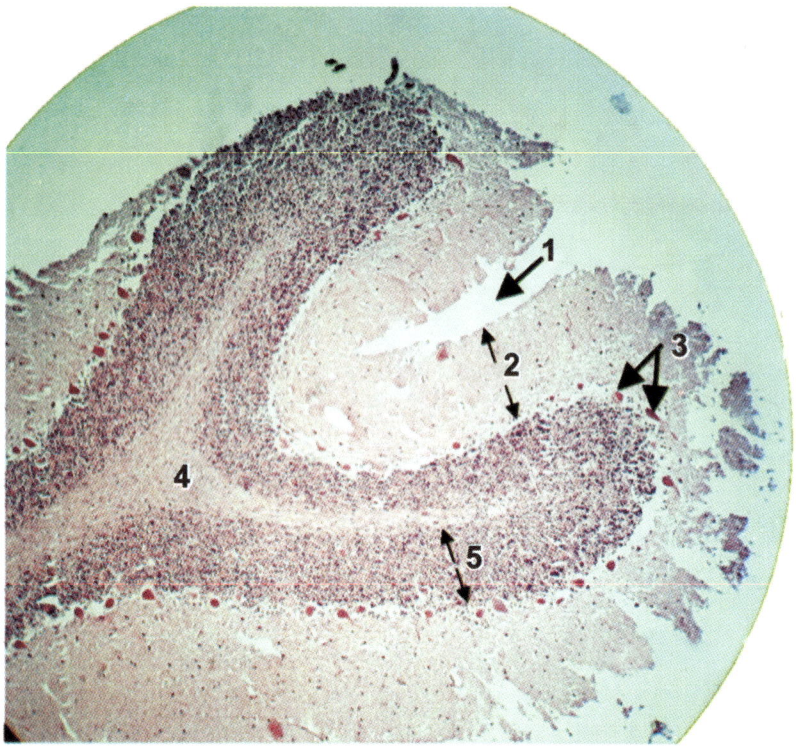

1. Interfolial sulcus
2. Cortex: Molecular layer (outer)
3. Purkinje cells
4. White matter
5. Cortex: Granular layer (inner)

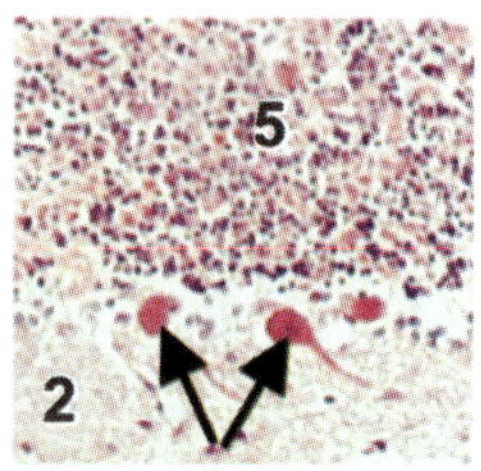

Key Features to Identify the Slide

- Outermost molecular cell layer
- Middle Purkinje cell layer
- Inner granular cell layer
- Presence of white matter in medulla

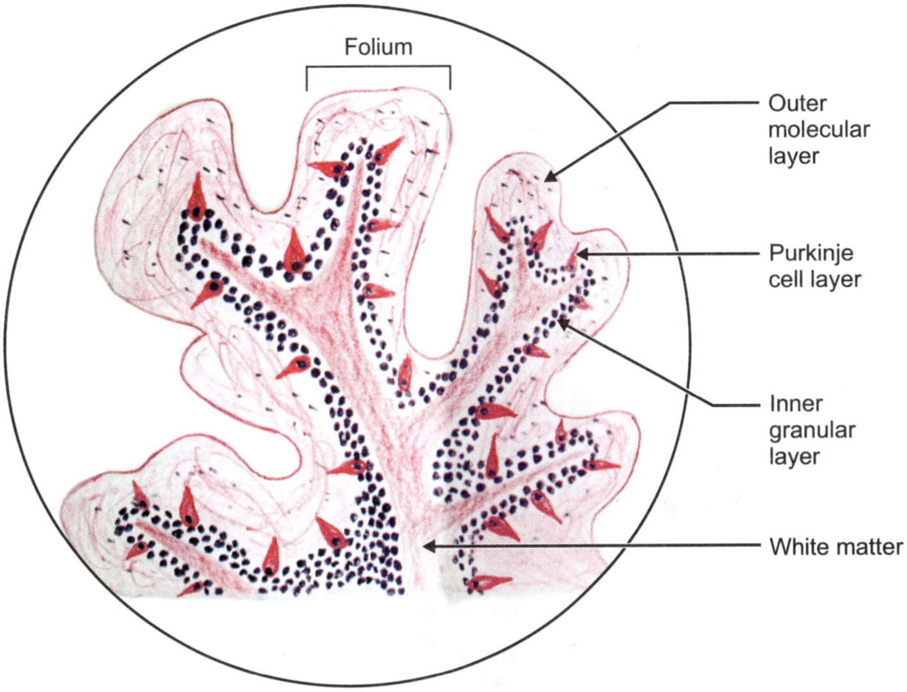
Folium
Outer molecular layer
Purkinje cell layer
Inner granular layer
White matter

SPINAL CORD: TRANSVERSE SECTION (TS)

The transverse section of spinal cord exhibits H-shaped gray matter in the centre surrounded by white matter.

Gray matter: Consists of pair of ventral (anterior) and dorsal (posterior) horns made up of large-sized multipolar motor neurons. In the central part, there is a central canal lined by ependymal cells made up of a layer of ciliated columnar epithelium.

In the thoracic region gray matter consists of lateral horns.

White matter: It is organised into anterior (ventral), lateral and posterior (dorsal) funiculi. It is made up of axons of ascending and descending tracts (myelinated nerve fibres).

Spinal cord is covered from outside to inside by three meningeal layers—dura mater, arachnoid mater and pia mater.

Applied Aspects of Central Nervous System

1. Multiple sclerosis: Myelinated nerve fibres of brain and spinal cord are progressively damaged due to destruction of myelin sheath resulting in blindness, sensory loss and muscular weakness.
2. Motor neuron disease: Degenerative disorder of motor neurons affecting ventral horn of spinal cord, upper motor neuron of corticospinal tract which manifests as asymmetrical weakness of limbs.

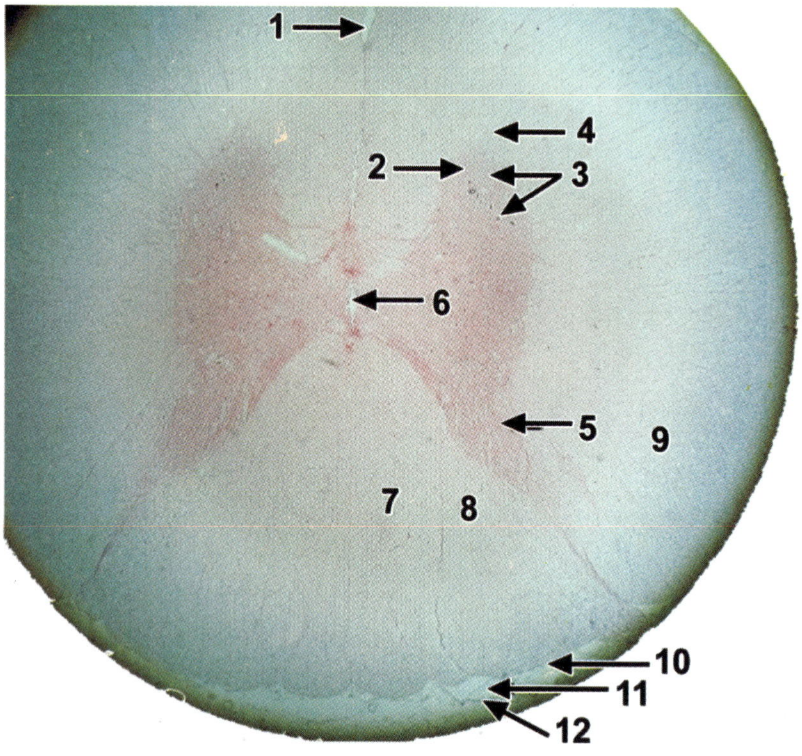

1. Anterior median fissure
2. Anterior gray horn
3. Anterior gray horn with motor neurons
4. Axons of anterior root
5. Posterior gray horn
6. Central canal
7. Fasciculus gracilis
8. Fasciculus cuneatus
9. Lateral white column
10. Pia mater
11. Subarachnoid space
12. Arachnoid

(7 and 8: Posterior white column)

Key Features to Identify the Slide

- H-shaped gray matter in the centre
- Presence of central canal lined by ependymal cells
- Gray matter surrounded by white matter

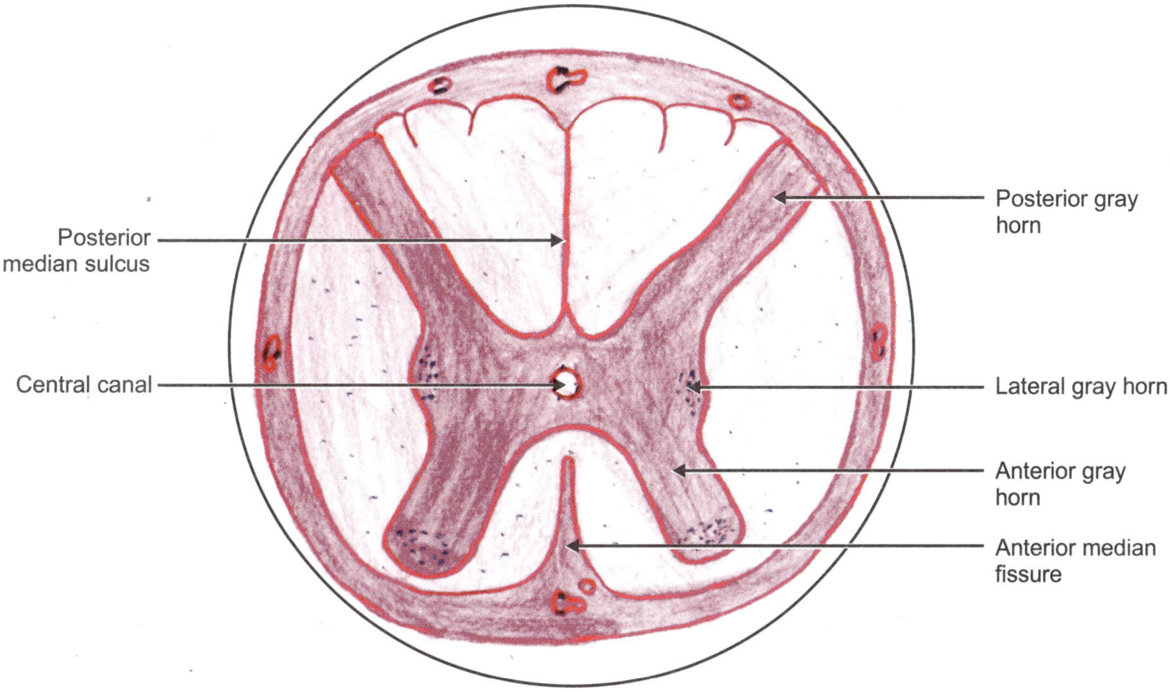
Posterior median sulcus
Central canal
Posterior gray horn
Lateral gray horn
Anterior gray horn
Anterior median fissure

QUESTIONS

1. Discuss and describe the layers of the cerebral cortex, including the various types of cells present in each layer. 5M
2. Name the neurons present in different layers of the cerebellar cortex. 2M
3. Explain the internal features of the spinal cord. 5M
4. What are climbing fibers. 2M
5. Explain the structure of Purkinje cells. 2M

Figures/Notes

THICK SKIN

Epidermis: Made up of stratified squamous keratinized epithelium arranged in 5 layers from deep to superficial as follows:

(a) Stratum basale/basal layer—consists of a single layer of columnar/cuboidal cells that exhibits high mitotic activity replenishing the cells in the superficial layer.

(b) Stratum spinosum/prickle cell layer—made up of several layers of polygonal cells (keratinocytes). Held together by desmosomes. The cells tend to shrink during tissue processing except where they are joined by desmosomes, which give them their characteristic spiny appearance.

(c) Stratum granulosum/granular layer—made up of three to four layers of flattened cells. The cytoplasm of the cells contains numerous keratohyalin granules. They form an important component of the permeability barrier of the epidermis rendering it relatively waterproof.

(d) Stratum lucidum/clear layer—found only in thick skin. This eosinophilic layer is more reflective optically and contains nuclear debris. The cells contain compacted keratin filaments.

(e) Stratum corneum/cornified layer—consists of closely packed layers of dead keratinized flattened cells. This layer is final product of epidermal differentiation or cornification.

Dermis: Made up of connective tissue divided into two layers:

(a) Papillary layer—consists of loose connective tissue and shows finger-like projections called dermal papillae.

(b) Reticular layer—made up of dense irregular connective tissue, dermis is vascular and has rich supply of nerve fibres.

Thick skin being present in the region of palms and soles contains plenty of sweat glands but is devoid of hair follicles and sebaceous glands.

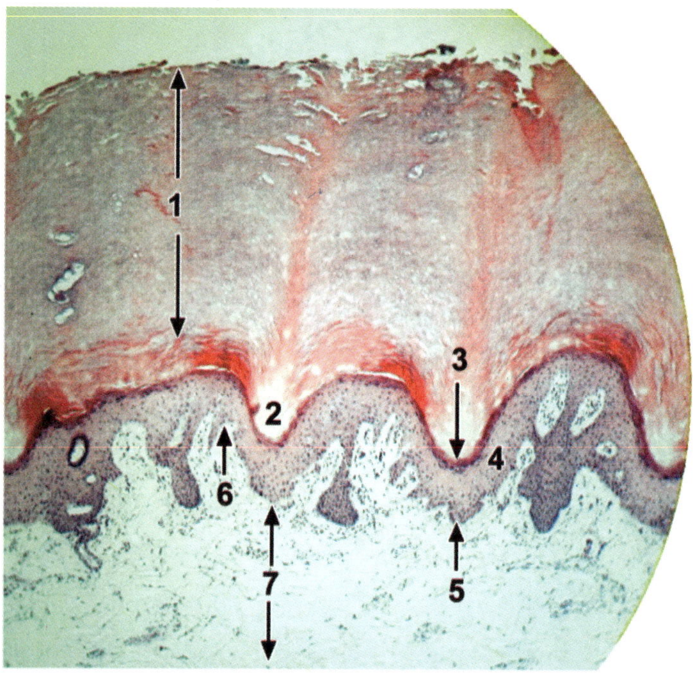

1. Stratum corneum
2. Stratum lucidum
3. Stratum granulosum
4. Stratum spinosum
5. Stratum basale
6. Dermal papillae
7. Dermis

Key Features to Identify the Slide

- Thick layer of epidermis lined by stratified squamous keratinized epithelium
- Prominent dermal and epidermal papillae
- Sweat glands are present
- Absence of hair follicles

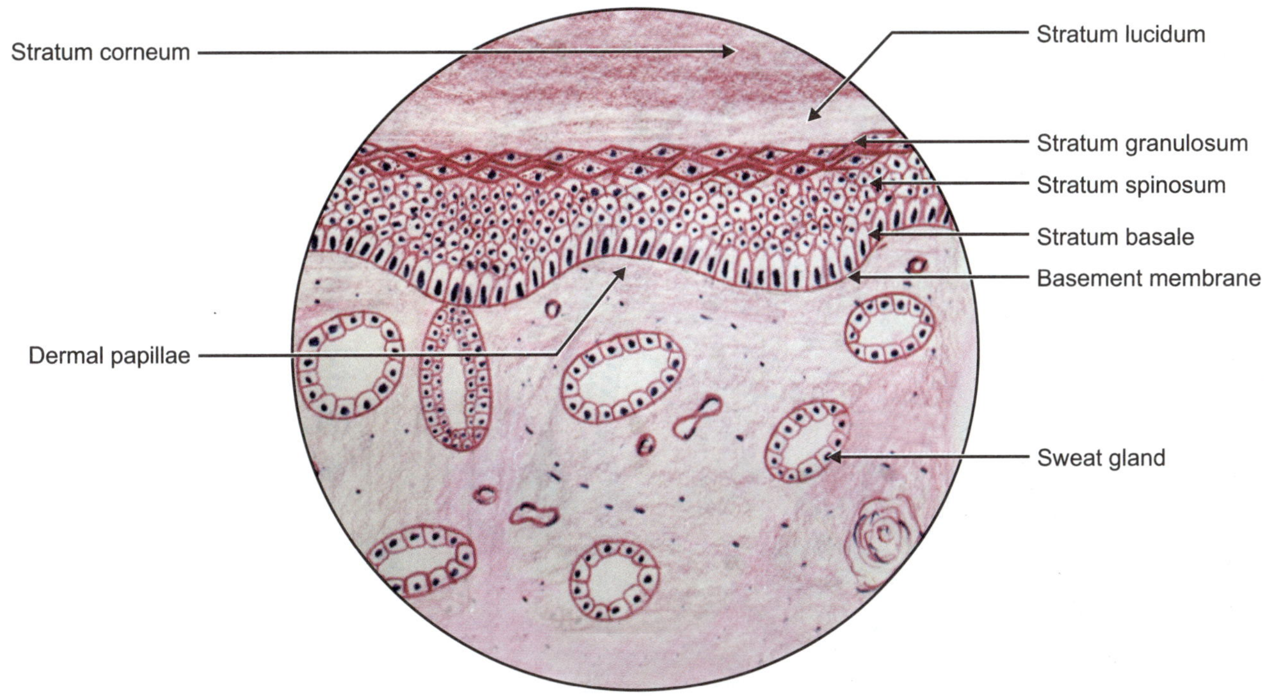
Stratum corneum
Stratum lucidum
Stratum granulosum
Stratum spinosum
Stratum basale
Basement membrane
Dermal papillae
Sweat gland

THIN SKIN

Epidermis: Made up of stratified squamous keratinized epithelium.

Among all its layers stratum lucidum is absent in thin skin. Stratum spinosum and stratum corneum are thin.

Dermis: Made up of connective tissue but does not show dermal papilla. Thin skin is present in all parts of the body except palms and soles. It contains hair follicles, arrector pili muscle, and sebaceous glands but few sweat glands.

Applied Aspects of Integumentary System

1. Vitiligo: Patchy depigmentation of skin due to degeneration and disappearance of melanocytes.
2. Basal cell carcinoma: One of the most common skin tumors in adults arising from basal cells occurring because of chronic exposure to ultraviolet radiation.

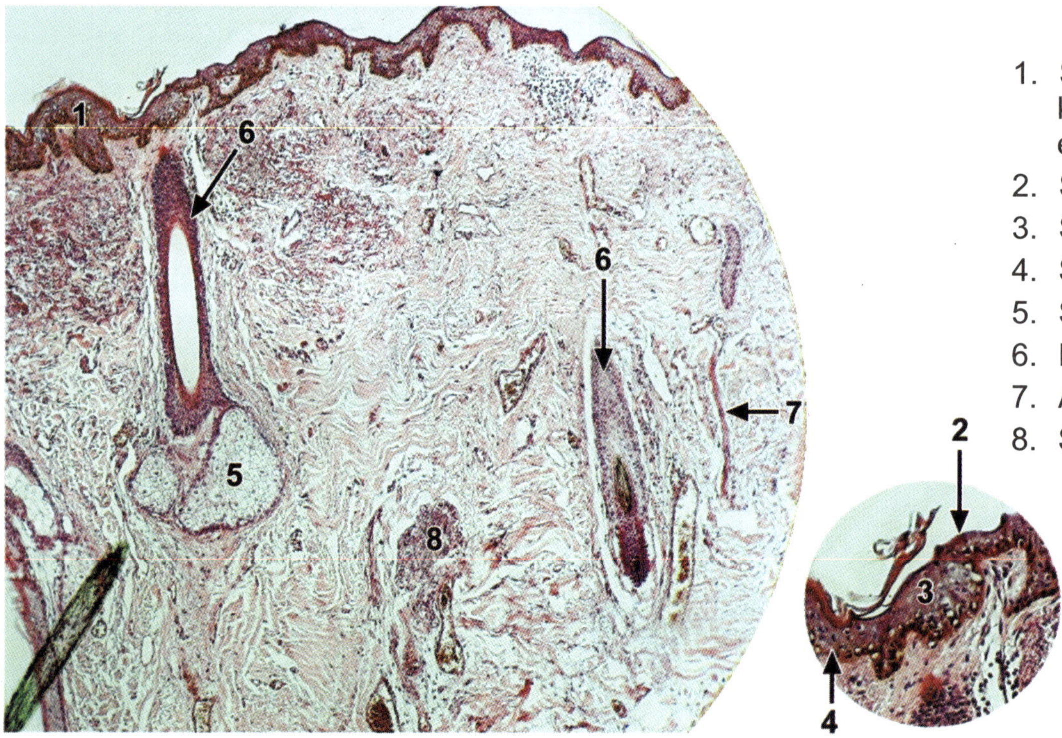

1. Stratified squamous keratinized epithelium
2. Stratum corneum
3. Stratum spinosum
4. Stratum basale
5. Sebaceous gland
6. Hair follicles
7. Arrector pili
8. Sweat gland

Key Features to Identify the Slide

- Thin layer of epidermis lined by stratified squamous keratinized epithelium
- Presence of hair follicles and sebaceous glands
- Presence of arrector pili muscle

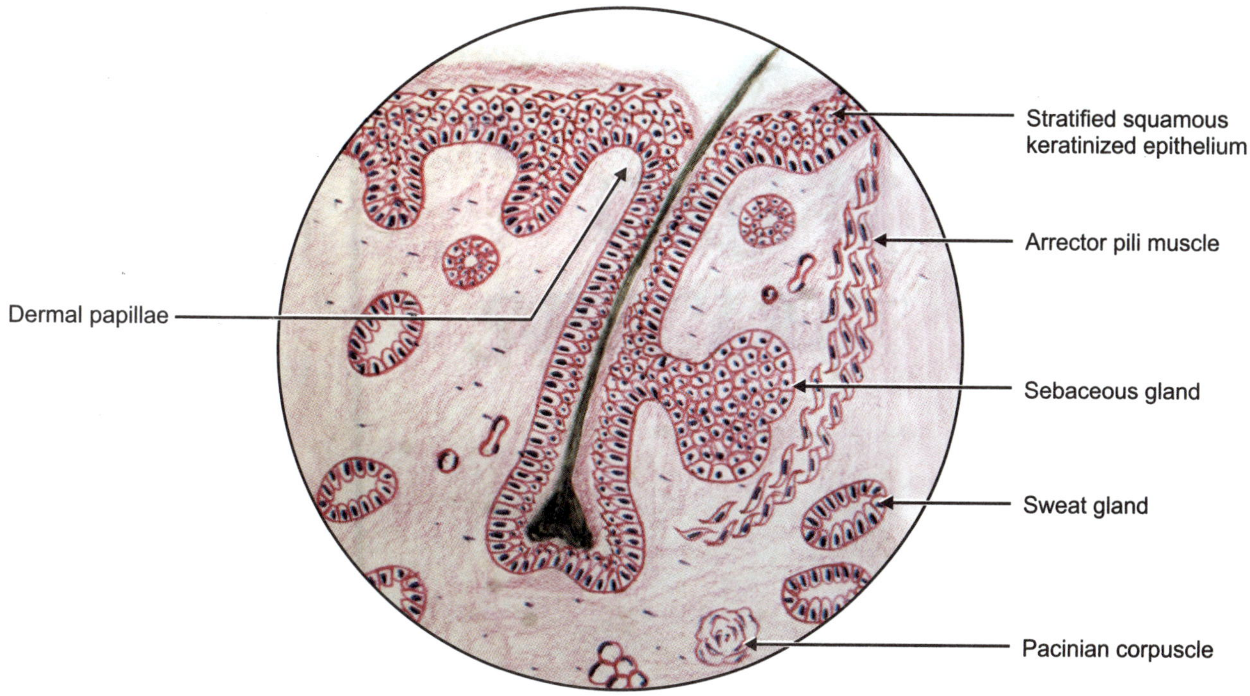
Stratified squamous keratinized epithelium
Arrector pili muscle
Dermal papillae
Sebaceous gland
Sweat gland
Pacinian corpuscle

QUESTIONS

1. Compare the microscopic features of thick skin and thin skin. 5M
2. Enumerate the layers of the epidermis. 2M
3. Describe the mode of secretion of apocrine sweat glands. 2M
4. List the different layers of the dermis. 2M
5. Define the pilosebaceous apparatus. 2M
6. Categorize sweat glands with examples. 2M

Figures/Notes

20 Organ of Special Senses (AN 43.2, 43.3)

EYELID

1. Outer surface lined by skin containing hair follicles with associated sebaceous glands of Zeis and sweat glands of Moll.
2. Deep to the skin is the skeletal muscle layer made up of orbicularis oculi muscle.
3. Presence of tarsal plate made up of dense collagenous connective tissue with specialized sebaceous glands embedded in it called tarsal (Meibomian) glands.
4. Internal surface lined by palpebral conjunctiva made up of stratified columnar epithelium.

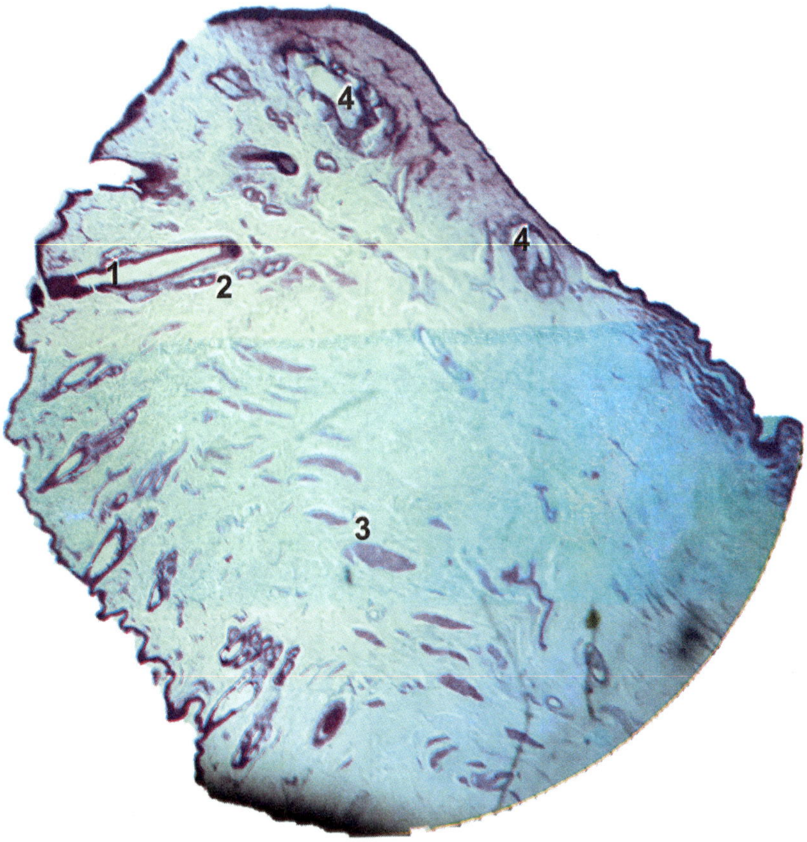

1. Hair follicle
2. Sebaceous gland
3. Orbicularis oculi
4. Tarsal gland

Key Features to Identify the Slide

- External surface covered by skin
- Internal surface covered by palpebral conjunctiva
- Presence of skeletal muscle and tarsal plate in between the two surfaces

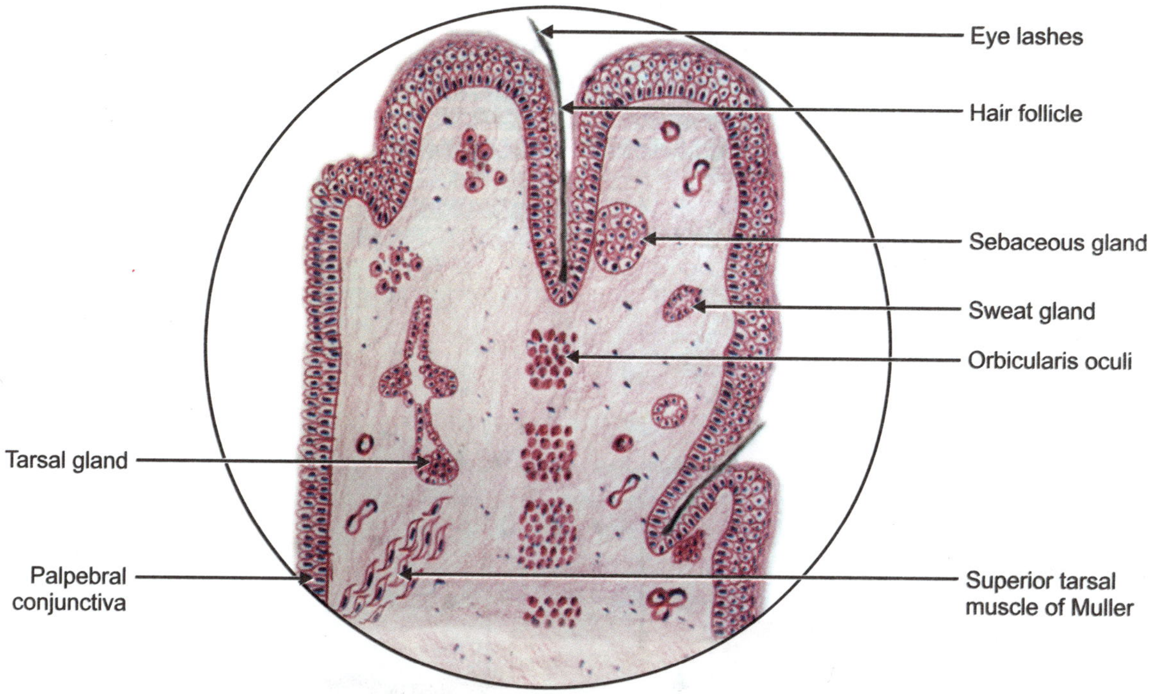
Eye lashes
Hair follicle
Sebaceous gland
Sweat gland
Orbicularis oculi
Tarsal gland
Palpebral conjunctiva
Superior tarsal muscle of Muller

CORNEA

Consists of five layers arranged from superficial to deep as follows:

1. Corneal epithelium—lined by stratified squamous non-keratinized epithelium, containing 5–6 layers of cells. It is protective in nature.
2. Anterior limiting membrane (Bowman's layer)—it is made up of dense mass of collagen fibrils which is amorphous in nature.
3. Substantia propria (stroma)—this layer forms the bulk of the cornea; it is compact and transparent being composed of 200 to 250 lamellae of parallel fibrils of type I collagen. The nuclei of flattened fibroblasts are located in between the lamellae.
4. Posterior limiting membrane (Descemet's layer)—it is thin homogeneous and is considered as basement membrane of endothelium.
5. Endothelium—consists of single layer of squamous cells covering the posterior surface of cornea.

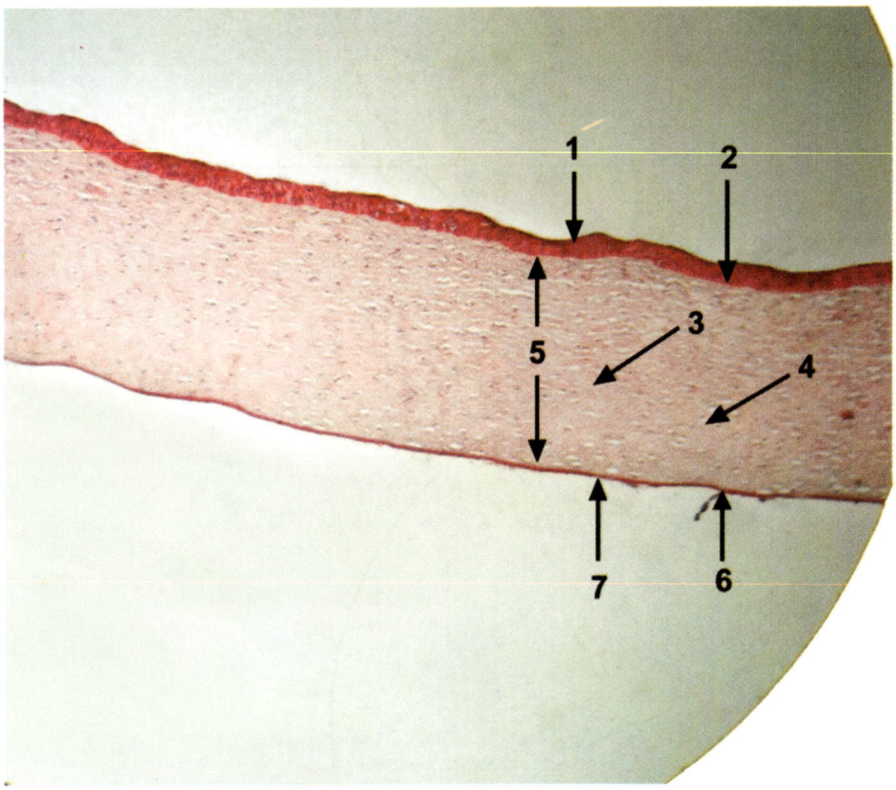

1. Stratified squamous non-keratinized epithelium
2. Anterior limiting (Bowman's) membrane
3. Nucleus of fibroblast
4. Collagen fibre
5. Corneal stroma (substantia propria)
6. Posterior limiting (Descemet's) membrane
7. Posterior epithelium (simple cuboidal)

Key Features to Identify the Slide

- Stratified squamous non-keratinized epithelium
- Bundles of collagen fibres with fibroblasts in substantia propria
- Inner layer of endothelium

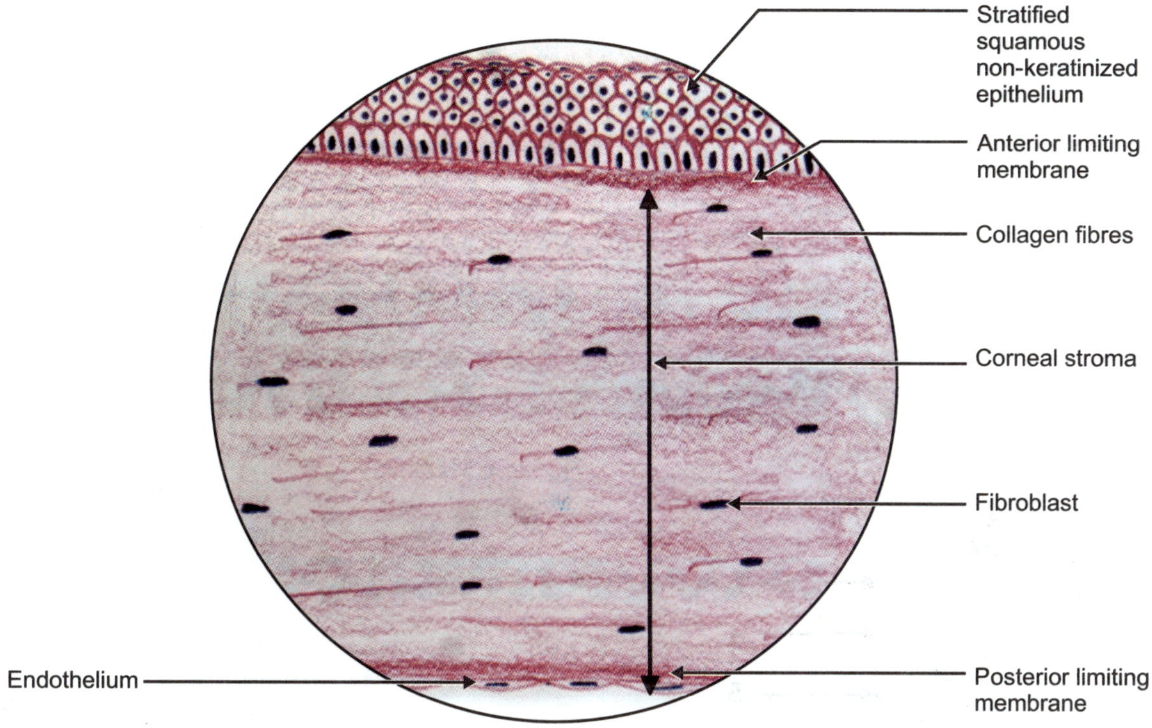
Stratified squamous non-keratinized epithelium
Anterior limiting membrane
Collagen fibres
Corneal stroma
Fibroblast
Endothelium
Posterior limiting membrane

RETINA

Consists of following layers from outside as follows:

1. Pigment epithelium—composed of a single layer of cuboidal cells, their cytoplasm contains numerous melanosomes and apically the cells bear long microvilli, which project between the outer segment of rods and cones.
2. Layer of rods and cones—this layer consists of photoreceptors, rods and cones. The outer segment of the cones are thicker and cone-shaped, whereas that of rod cells are cylindrical.
3. Outer limiting membrane—it is formed by processes of glial cells called as Muller cells.
4. Outer nuclear layer—consists of nuclei of rods and cones.
5. Outer plexiform layer—made up of axons of rods and cones which synapse with the dendrites of bipolar cells.
6. Inner nuclear layer—made up of cell bodies of bipolar cells, amacrine cells, horizontal cells and Müller cells.
7. Inner plexiform layer—consists of axons of bipolar cells which synapse with the dendrites of ganglion cells and amacrine cells.
8. Ganglion cell layer—consists of large cell bodies of ganglion cells and their axon forms optic nerve.
9. Nerve fibre layer—consists of axons of ganglion cells which travel towards the optic disc as optic nerve.
10. Inner limiting membrane—made up of processes of Müller cells.

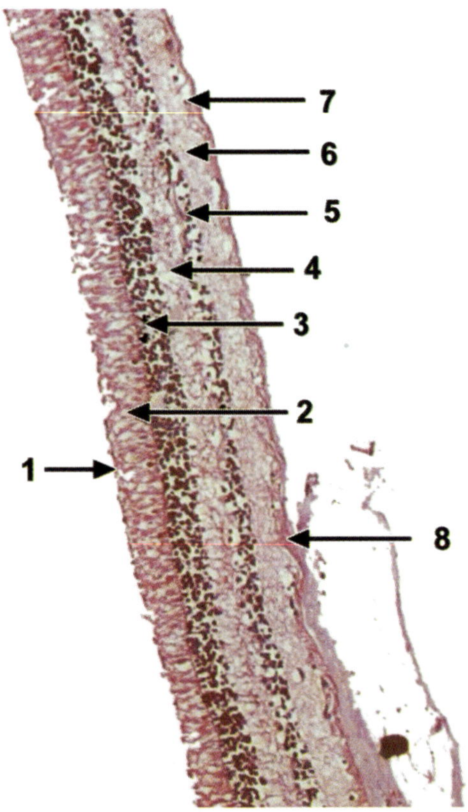

1. Pigment epithelium
2. Layer of rods and cones
3. Outer nuclear layer
4. Outer plexiform layer
5. Inner nuclear layer
6. Inner plexiform layer
7. Ganglion cell layer
8. Optic nerve fibre layer

Key Features to Identify the Slide

- Pigment cell layer—outermost
- Presence of rods and cones
- Presence of ganglionic cell layer

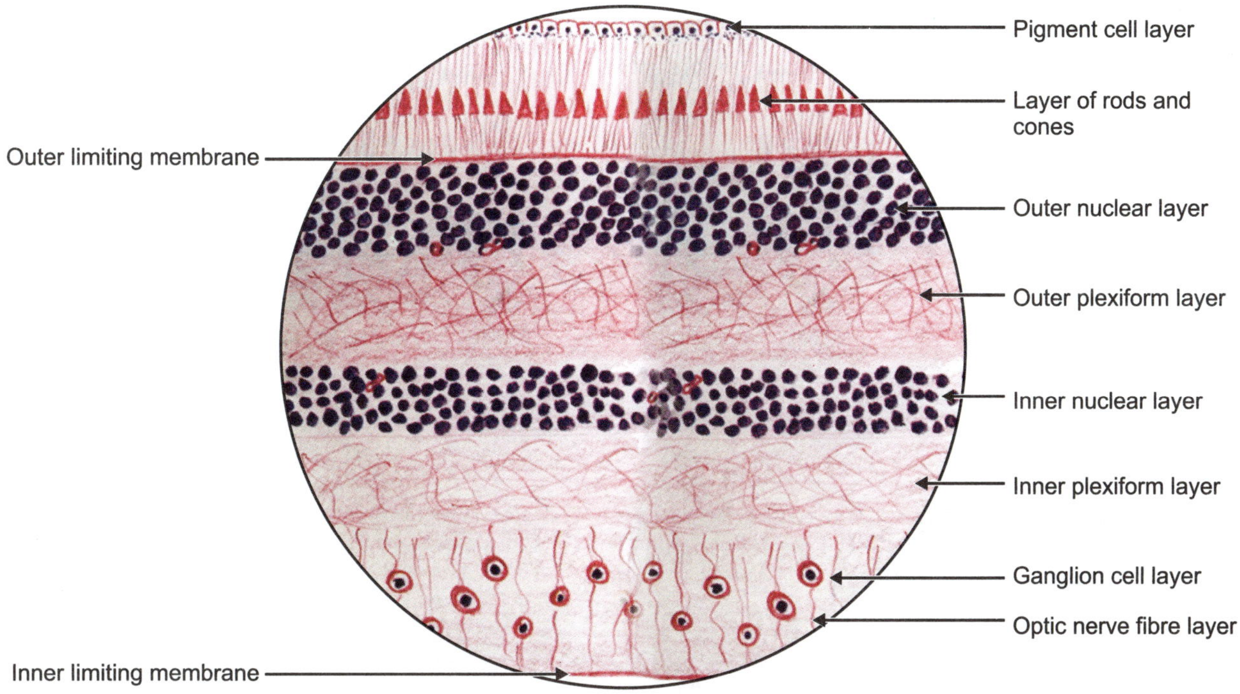
Pigment cell layer
Layer of rods and cones
Outer limiting membrane
Outer nuclear layer
Outer plexiform layer
Inner nuclear layer
Inner plexiform layer
Ganglion cell layer
Optic nerve fibre layer
Inner limiting membrane

OPTIC NERVE: TRANSVERSE SECTION (TS)

Transverse section of optic nerve shows following features—covered by three layers of meninges: Outer dura mater, middle arachnoid mater, and inner pia mater.

From the pia mater numerous septa arise and divide the interior of optic nerve into a number of fascicles.

Central artery and vein of retina is prominently visible in the central region of section of optic nerve.

Applied Aspects of Organ of Special Senses

1. Corneal opacity: Following injury, there occurs disruption of epithelial layer and stroma of cornea.
2. Retinal detachment: The nervous layer of retina gets separated from the pigment layer leading to blindness.

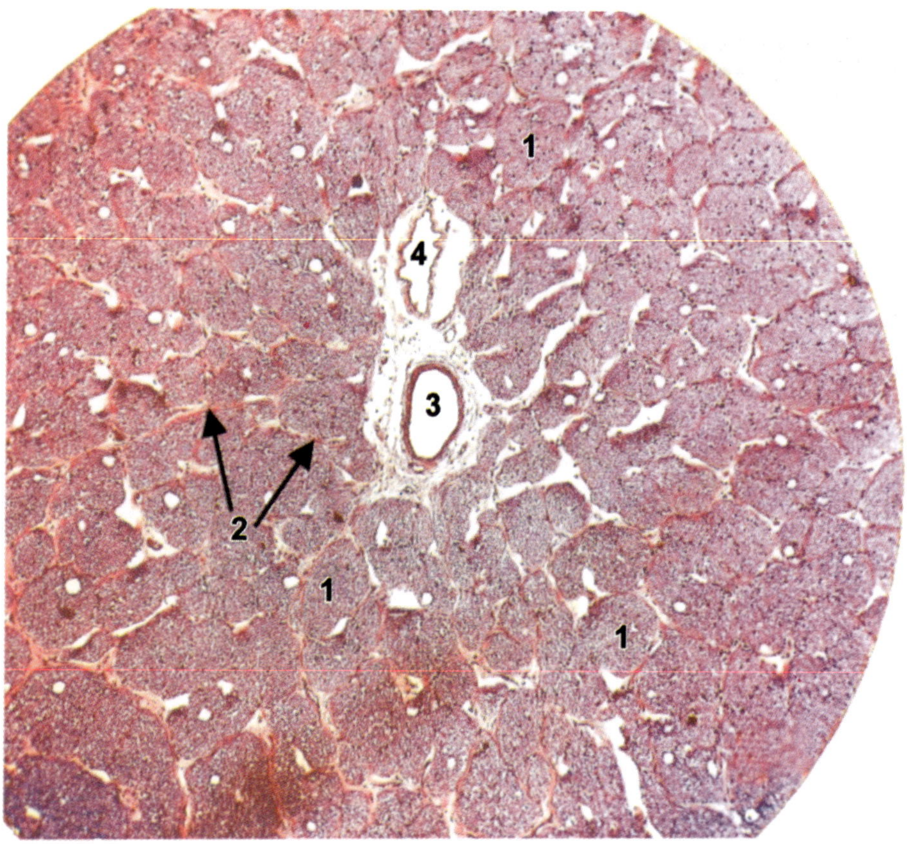

1. Bundles of optic nerve fibres
2. Pial sheaths
3. Central artery of retina
4. Central vein of retina

Key Features to Identify the Slide

- Presence of bundles of myelinated axons
- Presence of central artery and central vein of retina in the centre
- Three meningeal layers are seen—dura mater, arachnoid mater and pia mater

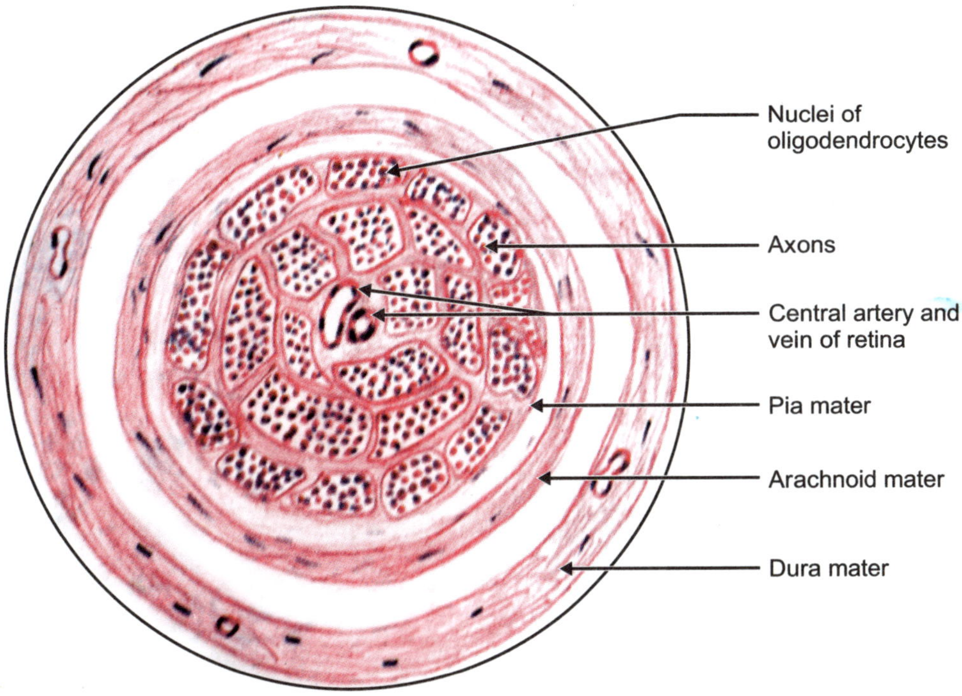
Nuclei of oligodendrocytes
Axons
Central artery and vein of retina
Pia mater
Arachnoid mater
Dura mater

QUESTIONS

1. Enumerate the layers of the retina and mention the different types of cells present in each layer. 5M
2. List the layers constituting the eyelid. 2M
3. Compare the structure and functions of rods and cones. 5M
4. Enumerate the layers of cornea and provide a brief description of the composition of each layer. 5M
5. Microanatomy of optic nerve. 5M
6. What are Müller cells. 2M

Figures/Notes